JN050509

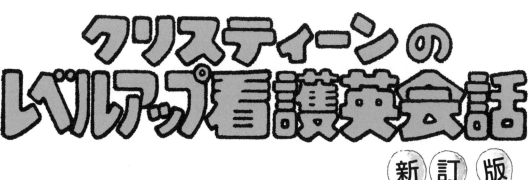

クリスティーンのレベルアップ看護英会話

新訂版

知念クリスティーン
元九州大学助教授

迫　和子

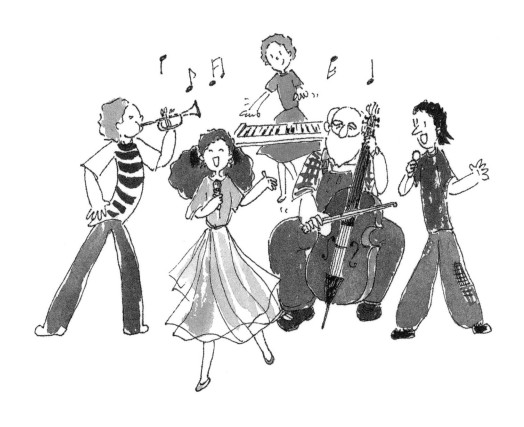

医学書院

略歴

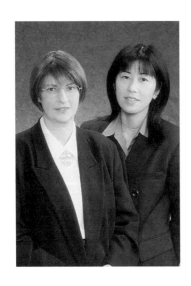

知念 クリスティーン リー（Christine Lee Chinen）

ニューヨーク市立大学にて教育学修士号と数学士号を取得.
日本で 21 年間英語を教える. 元九州大学大学教育研究セン
ター助教授. 医学英語を専門とする. 著書—『クリスティー
ンのやさしい看護英会話』（医学書院），『English-Live！』
(Intercom Press) をはじめ論文多数.
『クリスティーンのレベルアップ看護英会話』の初版は台湾，
韓国でも翻訳出版されている.

迫 和子（Kazuko Sako）

西南学院大学大学院博士前期課程修了（英文学）. 国立南福
岡病院附属高等看護学校，福岡女子短期大学，西南学院大学
各校の非常勤講師を経て現在翻訳業. The Economist 誌をは
じめ医学・英語学関係の翻訳および英検，バイリンガル教育，
英語教育法の研究に携わる. 著書—『ロッタとハナの楽しい
基本看護英語』（共著，医学書院），訳書—H. R. パッチ『異界
—中世ヨーロッパの夢と幻想』（共訳，三省堂），同『中世文
学における運命の女神』（共訳，三省堂）など.

クリスティーンのレベルアップ**看護英会話**

発　行　2001 年 10 月 15 日　第 1 版第 1 刷
　　　　2022 年 11 月 1 日　第 1 版第 20 刷
　　　　2023 年 11 月 1 日　新訂版第 1 刷ⓒ

著　者　知念クリスティーン・迫 和子

発行者　株式会社　医学書院
　　　　代表取締役　金原　俊
　　　　〒113-8719　東京都文京区本郷 1-28-23
　　　　電話　03-3817-5600（社内案内）

印刷・製本　アイワード

本書の複製権・翻訳権・上映権・譲渡権・貸与権・公衆送信権（送信可能化権
を含む）は株式会社医学書院が保有します.

ISBN978-4-260-05251-1

本書を無断で複製する行為（複写，スキャン，デジタルデータ化など）は，「私
的使用のための複製」など著作権法上の限られた例外を除き禁じられています.
大学，病院，診療所，企業などにおいて，業務上使用する目的（診療，研究活
動を含む）で上記の行為を行うことは，その使用範囲が内部的であっても，私的
使用には該当せず，違法です. また私的使用に該当する場合であっても，代行
業者等の第三者に依頼して上記の行為を行うことは違法となります.

[JCOPY]〈出版者著作権管理機構 委託出版物〉
本書の無断複製は著作権法上での例外を除き禁じられています.
複製される場合は，そのつど事前に，出版者著作権管理機構
（電話 03-5244-5088，FAX 03-5244-5089，info@jcopy.or.jp）の
許諾を得てください.

謝辞

　本書の出版にあたり多くの方々にさまざまな形でお世話になりました。井上博雅先生，甲斐貞子先生，佐藤昌司先生，浜田雄蔵先生，宮崎亮先生，西恵美子氏，松石貴子氏，June Seat 氏，Margaret Cane 氏，Monica Hellman 氏からは医学関係の知識など有益な情報をいただきました。済生会福岡総合病院院長の岡留健一郎先生をはじめ，病棟看護師の皆様には，医療現場からの貴重なご意見をいただきました。ここに改めて感謝申し上げます。

　また適切なアドバイスとご助力をいただいた医学書院編集部の方々，そして支え励ましてくれた家族にも，心からお礼を述べたいと思います。

2001 年 9 月

知念クリスティーン

迫　和子

新訂版に添えて

　初版発行以来，本書を活用していただいた多くの皆様に感謝申し上げます。おかげさまで今回，時流に合わせて内容を改めた新訂版を制作し，合わせて電子版も発行することができました。初版を作ったとき，少しでもよいものをお届けしようと，たくさんの苦労と楽しみを分かち合った知念クリスティーンと共に喜びたいと思います。

　近年，医学は驚くほどの進歩を遂げていますが，それでもなお医療現場は新たな困難に直面し続けています。その中で真摯な努力を続けておられる医療関係者の皆様と，その現場に加わるために研鑽の日々を送っておられる学生の皆様に，本書が少しでもお役に立てますよう心から願っています。

　初版からずっと本書を見守り育ててくださった，編集部の藤居尚子様をはじめ医学書院の皆様に厚く御礼申し上げます。

2023 年 10 月

迫　和子

Introduction

I am an American who has lived in Japan for 21 years. While living in Japan I have often had to visit a hospital both because of my children and for myself. Visiting a hospital has given me many chances to talk with nurses.

When talking with nurses in Japanese hospitals, I have encountered many who experience considerable frustration at not being able to communicate adequately with their foreign patients. Some nurses told me they could not give even simple instructions; other nurses spoke of wanting to be able to reassure patients about their treatment or disease.

On the other hand, foreigners who find themselves in a Japanese hospital often experience anxiety at not knowing what is going to happen to them. It is usually possible to find an English-speaking doctor in any specialty. However, if a person is admitted to the hospital, then merely having an English-speaking doctor will probably not be sufficient. While the doctor's daily visit usually lasts only a few minutes, it is the nurses who spend 24 hours a day caring for the patient. It is to help nurses and English-speaking foreign patients communicate that I have written two conversation textbooks for nurses.

This book is intended for students who have completed my first book, *Christine's Easy English Conversation for Nurses* or those who are at a pre-intermediate or intermediate level of English.

This book has been designed to be used either in a classroom with a teacher or individually by yourself. Except for the game, all the activities can be done by yourself using the book and audio tracks. If you are studying the book on your own, you can write a dialog when doing the role play activity (instead of speaking with a partner). In the back of the textbook, there is a handy glossary containing the difficult vocabulary in the book, and a section containing the listening practice transcripts and answers to other exercises.

Studying this book will help you develop the skills to communicate with your patients. Even if your English is not perfect, your patients will appreciate your efforts to speak their language. After studying this book you will be able to ask patients questions to get information in order to care for them properly. In addition, you will be able to reassure patients by explaining their treatment and care.

There is another matter of critical importance when you are communicating with a patient. You must be sure that you understand exactly what the patient is saying since a misunderstanding could be fatal in a hospital setting. Therefore, I have provided a section called "Emergency English" in Unit 1 that you should memorize and use when speaking with your patient to make sure that you really do understand your patient's meaning. It is not only learners of a foreign language that should ask for clarification, but even among Japanese-Japanese or English-English speakers there are misunderstandings. It is not a sign of your lack of language ability if you have to ask for clarification, but rather a way to ensure proper medical care.

I hope that you will enjoy using this textbook. I encourage you to embark on the challenging, but rewarding journey of becoming a more effective English speaker.

April, 2001

Christine Lee Chinen

ネイティブスピーカーの発音は医学書院のウェブサイト
https://www.igaku-shoin.co.jp/book/detail/113475/appendix
からダウンロードできます.
ID：kangoeikaiwa2
PW：christine

CONTENTS

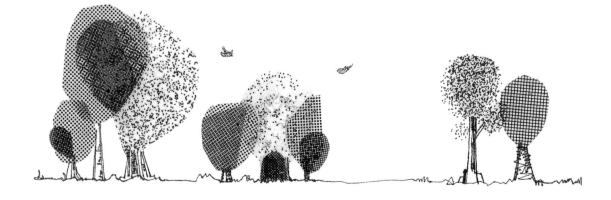

CONTENTS

表紙・本文イラスト：加藤　由美子

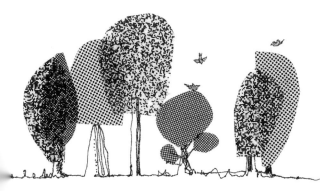
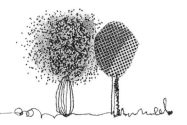

Do you work on the surgical ward ?

1 Listening Practice

Audio **2**

Listen to the conversations and choose the correct answers.

1. What is the woman's last name ?
   a) Delores   b) Argentina   c) Agosto

2. What is the man's phone number ?
   a) 03-4952-8614   b) 03-4952-8641   c) 03-4951-8614

3. What is the woman asking the man ?
   a) She wants to know his phone number.
   b) She wants to know his occupation.
   c) She wants to know what he is doing now.

4. What does Harvey Jones do ?
   a) He's an obstetrician.   b) He's a nurse.   c) He's a doctor.

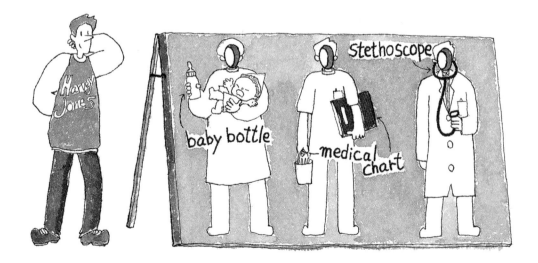

Emergency English ～困った時の英語～

イタリックの部分をほかの語に入れ替えて練習しましょう．

1. すみません，何と言ったのですか．（全文を聞き返す）
Excuse me ? ／ Pardon ?
Could you say that again, please ?

2. 13 ですか 30 ですか．（一部を聞き返す）
Did you say *thirteen* or *thirty* ?

3. もっとゆっくり話してもらえますか．
Could you speak more slowly ?

4. もっと大きな声で話してもらえますか．
Could you speak more loudly ?

5. すみません，わかりません．
I'm sorry, I don't understand.

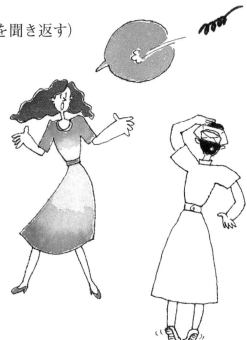

6. "X-ray technician" はどういう意味ですか．
What is the meaning of *X-ray technician* ?

7. それ（あなたの姓，名）はどう綴りますか．
How do you spell *that* ?
How do you spell your *family*（first）name ?

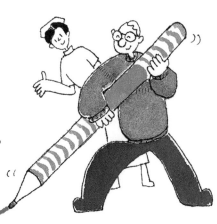

7

初対面のあいさつ

1. ややフォーマルな場合

Mary : *Sam*, this is *Frank Sawyer*. *Frank*, this is *Sam Hernandez.*
  Sam : How do you do ? It's nice to meet you.
Frank : It's nice to meet you, too.

2. ややくだけた場合

Mary : *Sam*, this is *Frank*. *Frank*, this is *Sam*.
  Sam : *Hello*〔Hi〕, it's nice to meet you.
Frank : Nice to meet you, too.

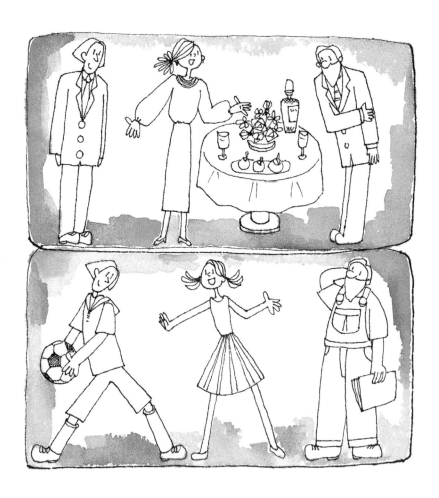

Listen to the dialog and fill in the missing words.

■ **Masako's First Day**

Head nurse : I want to 1)_____ you to some of the people you'll be working with. Masako, this is Dr. Kenichi Tanaka. He's the chief resident on this ward. Dr. Tanaka, this is Masako Sato. She's going to be working on this ward.

Masako : 2)_____, Dr. Tanaka. I'm very pleased to meet you.

Dr. Tanaka : I'm glad to meet you, too. 3)_____ to ask me about anything you don't understand.

Masako : I'll appreciate your help and patience until I get used to my job.

Dr. Tanaka : Well, I must continue my 4)_____ and see my patients.

Head nurse : We have 4 nurse's aides working here and there are 15 nurses and 6 doctors assigned to this ward. There's also a receptionist who does clerical work. I'll introduce you later. Let me bring you to the 5)_____ and you can meet the nurses who are coming off this shift.

■ **In the Nurses' Lounge**

Head nurse : 6)_____ Masako Sato. She's going to be your colleague. I have some work to do, so please introduce yourselves to Masako.

Masako : I'm Masako Sato and I'm going to be working on this 7)_____. I'm very happy to meet you all. I know I'll have a lot of questions at first, so I hope you can show me the ropes.

Eli : Masako, I'm Eli Hasegawa, and these are Mariko Murata, Yoko Deguchi, Akari Fujii and Kenji Shibata. Of course we'll 8)_____. Please ask about anything you like.

9

Masako : Thank you. I'm really glad to meet everyone. I know I'll enjoy working with all of you.

Akari : We're glad to meet our new colleague.

Eli : Where 9) _____ , Masako ?

Masako : I'm from Kyushu. I've been working at a Red Cross Hospital in Nagasaki for 8 years. But I went to 10) _____ in Tokyo and want to live here again. Where are you from, Eli ?

Eli : Oh, I'm a native Tokyo-ite. Which nursing school did you attend ?

Masako : I went to the nursing school attached to the National Medical Center.

Eli : Oh, me too! I graduated 5 years ago so 11) _____ . Where do you live ?

Masako : I found an apartment 12) _____ . How about you ?

Eli : I live with my parents and younger brother in Shinjuku. What are your 13) _____ ?

Masako : Well, I like playing tennis and singing karaoke.

Eli : I like playing tennis, too. Let's play together sometime. And we all like singing karaoke. Let's go to karaoke on our holiday.

Yoko : How about going next Saturday after work ?

Mariko, Akari, Kenji : That's a 14) _____ !

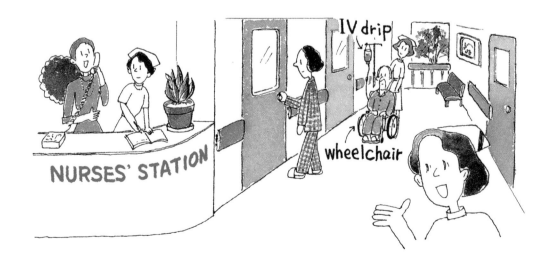

Department of...

internal medicine　内科

neurology　神経内科

cardiology　循環器内科

respiratory diseases　呼吸器内科

gastroenterology　消化器内科

psychosomatic medicine

心療内科

pediatrics　小児科

psychiatry　精神科

surgery　外科

orthopedics　整形外科

neurosurgery　脳神経外科

cardiosurgery　心臓外科

plastic surgery　形成外科

urology　泌尿器科

obstetrics/gynecology

産婦人科

dermatology　皮膚科

ophthalmology　眼科

oto (rhino) laryngology, ENT

耳鼻 (咽喉) 科

dentistry　歯科

oral surgery　口腔外科

radiology　放射線科

anesthesiology　麻酔科

rehabilitation　リハビリ科

Occupations

director of nursing　看護部長

head nurse　看護師長

chief nurse　主任看護師

nurse　看護師

nurse's aide　看護助手

student nurse　看護学生

midwife　助産師

doctor　医師

resident　レジデント，研修医

X-ray technician　放射線技師

lab technician　検査技師

CE (clinical engineer),

ME (medical engineer)

臨床工学技士

dietitian　栄養士

pharmacist　薬剤師

PT (physical therapist)

理学療法士

OT (occupational therapist)

作業療法士

ST (speech therapist)

言語聴覚士

dental hygienist　歯科衛生士

receptionist　受付

11

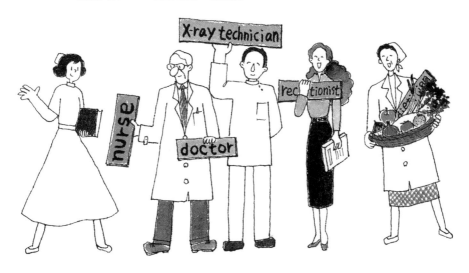

4 Activity Puzzle : Medical Occupations-Departments

私の職場はどこ？

下の職種の人はそれぞれ，どの診療科で働いているでしょうか．中央の文字列を並べ替え，正しい診療科名を右側の解答欄に書きましょう．

Job		Department
例) UROLOGIST	OYGLUOR	U R O L O G Y
1. MIDWIFE	ECSBTITOSR	1.
2. INTERNIST	ATNIENDECRNELIMI	2.
3. DENTAL HYGIENIST	TESINRDTY	3.
4. PEDIATRICIAN	DSEIITPACR	4.
5. X-RAY TECHNICIAN	RGOLAOIYD	5.
6. GYNECOLOGIST	EOYGYGOLNC	6.
7. CARDIOLOGIST	OCIRODALYG	7.
8. PLASTIC SURGEON	IRYTASPGUERCSL	8.
9. OPHTHALMOLOGIST	GOOLYLMPHTOAH	9.
10. PHYSICAL THERAPIST	BNAILOATIITEHR	10.
11. PSYCHIATRIST	SYYCPATHIR	11.
12. DERMATOLOGIST	OLAGREMTDYO	12.
13. ANESTHESIOLOGIST	HOLETGAOSEYSNI	13.
14. ORTHOPEDIST	IDRPHEOSTOC	14.
15. NEUROLOGIST	OYNRLEUOG	15.
16. ORAL SURGEON	ORYSAUGRLRE	16.

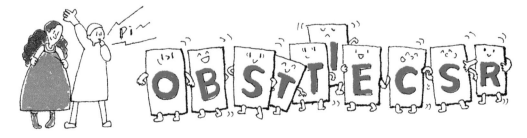

5 _{Activity} Role Play

患者の基本情報

　2人1組になり，看護師役(A)と患者役(B)を決め，カードの指示に従ってロールプレイをしましょう．下の書類は患者の基本情報を記入するためのものです．看護師役の人は患者役の人に質問して，書類に記入してください．終わったら役割を交替し，患者役(C)と看護師役(A)のカードを使って練習します．

　このロールプレイは必ず英語だけで行ってください．相手の言っていることが聞き取れなかったり，綴りなどがわからないときは，**Checkpoint** にある Emergency English を使いましょう．

Role Card A- Nurse

Your patient is a foreigner who can't speak Japanese.
Ask the patient questions to fill out the form.

氏名 ＿＿＿＿＿＿＿＿＿＿＿＿＿＿＿＿＿＿＿＿＿＿＿　性別 ＿＿＿＿＿＿

国籍 ＿＿＿＿＿＿＿＿＿＿＿　生年月日 ＿＿＿＿＿＿＿＿＿＿＿

既婚／未婚　　職業 ＿＿＿＿＿＿＿＿＿＿＿＿＿＿＿

住所 ＿＿＿＿＿＿＿＿＿＿＿＿＿＿＿＿＿＿＿＿＿＿＿

電話 (自宅・携帯) ＿＿＿＿＿＿＿＿＿　電話 (勤務先) ＿＿＿＿＿＿＿＿

家族構成 ＿＿＿＿＿＿＿＿＿＿＿＿＿＿＿＿＿＿＿＿

趣味 ＿＿＿＿＿＿＿＿＿＿＿＿＿＿＿＿＿＿＿＿＿＿

Role Card B - Patient ; Gerald Brown

Answer the nurse's questions, using the information below.

You are Irish. You were born in Dublin, Ireland on October 20, 1998. You are living with your girlfriend, Jenny. You are a dancer and a bartender. Your address is: Fujita Building #231, Yahatanishi-ku, Kitakyushu-shi, Fukuoka-ken, 807-0815. Your telephone number at home is: 093-845-3313 and at work is: 093-871-2487. Your hobbies are jogging and playing soccer.

Role Card C - Patient ; Mary Lee Smith

Answer the nurse's questions, using the information below.

You are American. You were born in Trenton, New Jersey, in the United States on August 13, 1992. You are married and have 3 children, 10-year-old twin sons and a 12-year-old daughter. You are a dental hygienist. Your address is: Grace Mansion #407, 3-1-55 Ropponmatsu, Chuo-ku, Osaka 541-0043. Your mobile phone number is: 090-0173-5222 and at work is: 06-7325-0880. Your hobbies are reading and knitting.

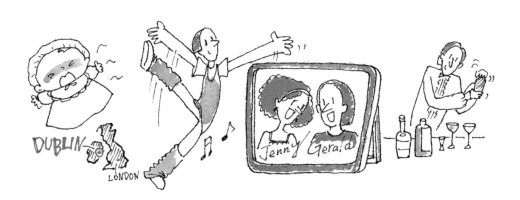

6 Activity Game : Name Game

どこまで覚えられる？

　このゲームでみんなの名前と趣味を覚えましょう．10〜15 人ずつのグループに分かれて輪になってください．最初の人が自分の名前と趣味を英語で言います．あとの人は自分より前の人の名前と趣味をすべて繰り返してから，最後に自分の名前と趣味を言ってください．

A : My name is Eli and my hobby is playing tennis.

B : Her name is Eli and her hobby is playing tennis.
　　My name is Taro and my hobby is riding a motorbike.

C : Her name is Eli and her hobby is playing tennis.
　　His name is Taro and his hobby is riding a motorbike.
　　My name is Sadako and my hobby is social dancing.

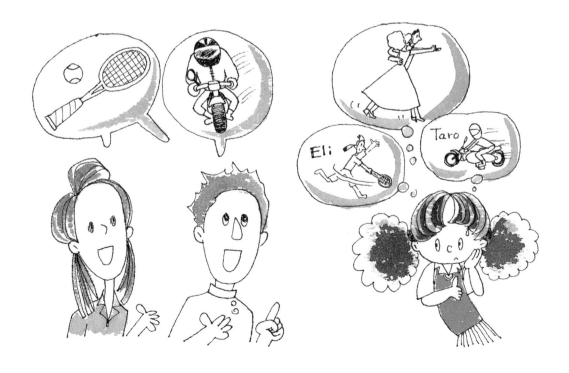

Unit 2 What's your problem today ?

1 Activity Listening Practice

Audio 5

Listen to the conversations and choose the correct answers.

1. What is wrong with the patient ?
   a) He doesn't have an insurance card.
   b) He's got lower back pain.
   c) He wants to go to the orthopedics department.

2. What are Mrs. Jefferson's symptoms ?
   a) She has constipation, a cough and a fever.
   b) She has a fever, diarrhea and a cough.
   c) She has diarrhea, lower back pain and a toothache.

16

3. Which department should the patient go to ?
   a) Plastic surgery   b) Surgery   c) Oral surgery

4. How long has Mr. Jones been having stomach pain ?
   a) For one week.   b) For two days.   c) For two months.

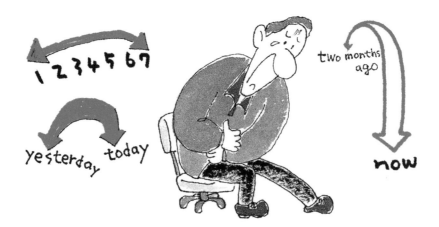

診療手続きをする

1. 前にこの病院にかかったことがありますか.

Have you visited this hospital before ?
Have you been a patient here before ?

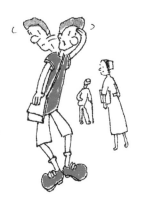

2. 診察券(保険証)をお持ちですか.

Do you have *this hospital's ID card* (an insurance card) ?

3. 何科にかかりたいのですか.

What department do you want to visit ?

4. この書類に記入してください.

Please fill *out* (in) this form.

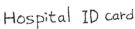

Hospital ID card

17

5. 身長(体重, 年齢)を教えてください.

Would you mind telling me your *height* (weight, age) ?
What is your *height* (weight, age) ?

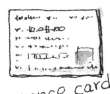
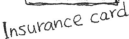
Insurance card

何歳ですか.

How old are you ?

身長はどのくらいですか.

How tall are you ?

体重はどのくらいですか.

How much do you weigh ?

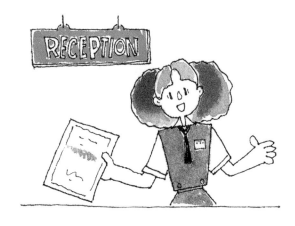

症状を尋ねる

1. どうしましたか.

What's your problem today ?
What seems to be the problem ?
What's the matter with you ?

2. どんなぐあいですか.

How have you been feeling ?

3. どんな症状ですか.

What are your symptoms ?

4. 症状はどれくらい(いつから)続いていますか.

How long have you had these symptoms ?
How long has this been going on ?

    3日間(週, 月)です.

    For 3 *days* (weeks, months).

    月曜日(先週, 先月)からです.

    Since *Monday* (last week, last month).

5. いつから嘔吐(咳)をしていますか.

How long have you *been vomiting* (had a cough) ?

6. 何回下痢をしましたか.

How many times did you have diarrhea ?

7. 熱はありますか.

Do you have a *fever* (temperature) ?

8. 熱は何度ですか.

What's your temperature ?

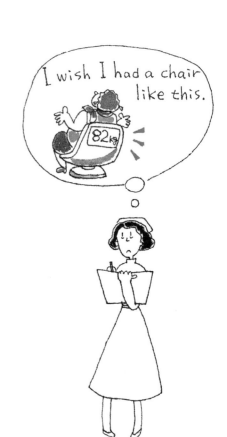

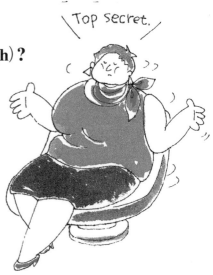

Measurement 測定の単位と略語

● 身長

ft	=	**foot, feet** フット，フィート	**1 ft = 12 in**
in	=	**inch** インチ	**1 in = 2.54 cm**
cm	=	**centimeter** センチ（メートル）	**1 cm = 0.394 in**

● 体重

lb	=	**pound** ポンド	**1 lb = 0.454 kg**
kg	=	**kilogram** キロ（グラム）	**1 kg = 2.2 lb**

● 体温

°F = Fahrenheit 華氏
°C = Celsius 摂氏
$$°F = °C × 1.8 + 32$$
$$°C = (°F - 32) ÷ 1.8$$

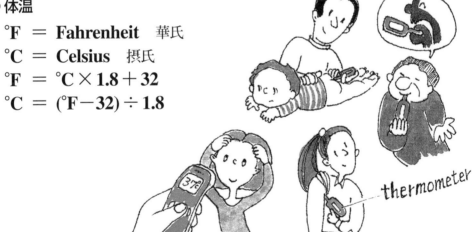

thermometer

> **Note** Some English-speaking countries still use Fahrenheit scale rather than Celsius. They use pounds, feet and inches, rather than kilograms, and centimeters.

3. Dialog

Listen to the dialog and fill in the missing words.

■ In the Outpatient Clinic

> **Masako** : Mr. Bergeron? Mr. Alexander Bergeron ?
>
> **Mr. Bergeron** : Yes?
>
> **Masako** : 1) _____ this hospital before ?
>
> **Mr. Bergeron** : Yes, I have. I was a patient here about 2 years ago.
>
> **Masako** : Do you have this hospital's ID card ?
>
> **Mr. Bergeron** : Yes, here it is.
>
> **Masako** : Can you 2) _____ ?
>
> **Mr. Bergeron** : I'm sorry, I can't read Japanese.
>
> **Masako** : OK, I'll fill it in for you. Now let me ask you some questions.
> 3) _____ your first and family names please ?
>
> **Mr. Bergeron** : Alexander is A-L-E-X-A-N-D-E-R and Bergeron is B-E-R-G-E-R-O-N.
>
> **Masako** : Thank you. OK, would you mind telling me your 4) _____ and weight ?
>
> **Mr. Bergeron** : I'm 175 cm tall and I 5) _____ 93 kg. I'm a little overweight.
>
> **Masako** : Could you tell me your age, please ?
>
> **Mr. Bergeron** : 6) _____ .
>
> **Masako** : Now, what is 7) _____ today ?
>
> **Mr. Bergeron** : I've been 8) _____ shortness of breath and some-times I experience a tightness in my chest and palpitations.
>
> **Masako** : 9) _____ has this been going on ?
>
> **Mr. Bergeron** : For 10) _____ weeks now.
>
> **Masako** : How often do you feel the tightness in your chest and palpitations ?

Mr. Bergeron : 11) _____ , especially when I exert myself — climb up stairs or walk very quickly.

Masako : Are you suffering any discomfort right now ?

Mr. Bergeron : No, I'm not.

Masako : Have you had any problems 12) _____ before ?

Mr. Bergeron : No, never.

Masako : Have you had any medical problems before ?

Mr. Bergeron : I had my gallbladder removed 13) _____ here before.

Masako : Do you have a fever ?

Mr. Bergeron : I don't know.

Masako : OK, let me take your temperature and your blood pressure. The doctor 14) _____ in a few minutes.

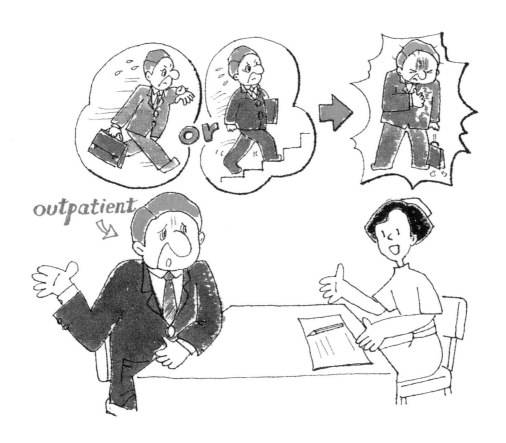

❤ Medical Terms : Symptoms - Usage

✎ I have...

a bloody nose　鼻血

bloody stools　血便

bloody urine　血尿

blurred vision　かすみ目

chills　悪寒

an eruption　発疹

eye discharge　目やに

a fever,　a temperature　熱

hiccups　しゃっくり

lesions　傷, 病変

a lump　腫れ物, しこり

no energy　無気力

a rash　発疹

a swelling　腫れ, こぶ

✎ I am suffering from...

appetite *loss* (gain)

　　　　　　食欲減退（増進）

constipation　便秘

convulsions　けいれん, ひきつけ

dizziness,　vertigo　めまい

excessive thirst　異常な喉の渇き

hearing loss　聴力喪失, 難聴

heat (cold) intolerance

　　　　　　熱（寒冷）不耐

incontinence　失禁

inflammation　炎症

lethargy　倦怠感

painful urination　排尿痛

weight *gain* (loss)

　　　　　　体重増加（減少）

✎ I have... /
　I am suffering from...

どちらにも使う語

abdominal pain　腹痛

a backache　背部（腰）痛

bloody stools　血便

chest pain　胸痛

a cough　咳

cramps　けいれん

diarrhea　下痢

an earache　耳痛

gas　おなら, ガス

a headache　頭痛

heartburn　胸やけ

heart flutters

　　　　（速く不規則な）動悸

insomnia　不眠（症）

joint pain　関節痛

lower back pain　腰痛

muscular aches　筋肉痛

nausea　吐き気

pain　痛み

palpitations　動悸（心悸亢進）

phlegm　痰

poor digestion　食欲不振

rapid heartbeat　動悸

a runny nose　鼻水

shortness of breath　息切れ

a sore throat　喉痛

a stiff *neck* (shoulders)

　　　　　　首（肩）の凝り

a stomachache　胃痛（腹痛）

a stuffy nose　鼻詰まり

a toothache　歯痛

an upset stomach　胃の不調

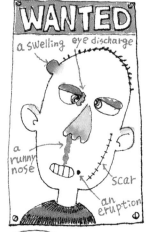

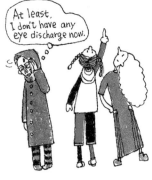

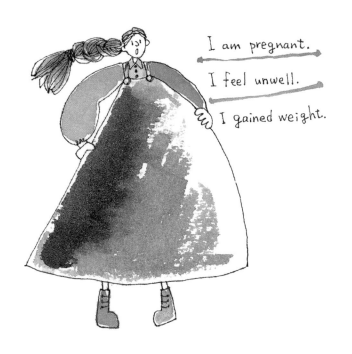

I am pregnant.
I feel unwell.
I gained weight.

✎ **I am... / I feel...**
どちらにも使う語

cranky　機嫌が悪い，むずかる

dizzy　めまいがする

gassy　ガスがたまった

itchy　かゆい

nauseous　吐き気がする

short of breath　息切れ(する)

sluggish　だるい

tired　疲れた

✎ **I...**

fainted　失神した

gained (lost) weight

　　　　　　太った(やせた)

vomited　嘔吐した

vomited blood　吐血した

23

✎ **I am...**

constipated　便秘している

coughing up blood

　　　　喀血がある

hard of hearing　難聴がある

having cold sweats

　　　冷汗をかいている

having seizures

　　　発作が起きている

pregnant　妊娠している

sneezing　くしゃみが出る

sweating　汗をかいている

vomiting　嘔吐している

vomiting blood　吐血している

wheezing　喘鳴がある

✎ **I feel...**

faint

　　ふらふらする，気を失いそう

lethargic　だるい，無気力な

numbness　しびれ

something stuck in my throat

　　　　　　喉の異物感

tightness in my chest

　　　胸が締めつけられる感じ

unwell　気分がよくない

weak　衰弱した，衰えた

✎ **My...**

leg is itchy　足がかゆい

back is painful

　　　　背中(腰)が痛い

right (left) side is numb

　　　　右(左)側がしびれている

finger is swollen

　　　　指が腫れている

toe is infected

　　　足の指が化膿している

4 Puzzle : Scrambled Sentences
Activity

ちぐはぐな会話

次の会話を正しい順番に並べ替えましょう．それぞれの文に番号をつけてください．

	Nurse : Do you have a fever ?
___	Patient : For 3 days.
___	Nurse : What's your problem today ?
___	Nurse : The doctor will see you in a few minutes.
___	Patient : I think I have a cold.
___	Nurse : How long have you had these symptoms ?
___	Patient : Yes, it is.
___	Patient : I have a cough and a headache.
1	Nurse : Is this your first visit ?
___	Patient : Yes, I do. My temperature is 38.2℃.
___	Nurse : What are your symptoms ?

24

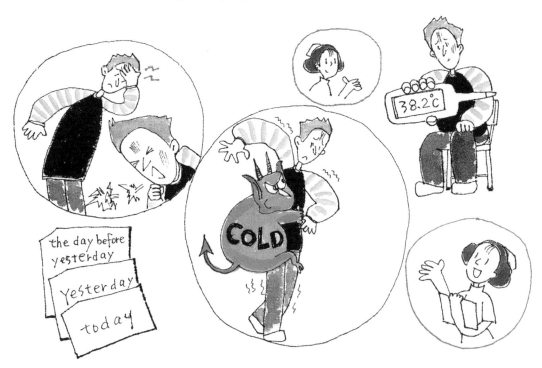

5 Role Play

Activity

診療申込書

2人1組になり，看護師役（A）と患者役（B）を決め，カードの指示に従ってロールプレイをしましょう．看護師は患者に質問して書類に記入してください．終わったら役割を交替して，患者役（C）と看護師役（A）のカードを使って練習します．

Role Card A - Nurse

Your patient is a foreigner who can't speak Japanese.
Ask the patient questions to fill in the form.

診療申込書

診療科：

内科　外科　産婦人科　整形外科　耳鼻咽喉科　眼科　リハビリ科　小児科

氏名 _____ **性別** _____

体重 _____ **身長** _____ **年齢** _____

どうしましたか：

どんな症状ですか：

いつ頃からですか：

何回くらいですか：

Role Card B - Patient；Alan Moss, 29-year-old male

You weigh 155 pounds and you are 5 feet 11 inches tall. You twisted your ankle when you were playing beach volleyball yesterday afternoon. Your ankle is very painful and swollen. You want to go to the orthopedic department.

Role Card C - Patient；Sandra Philips, 52-year-old female

You weigh 138 lb and are 5 ft 6 in tall. You have pain in your right abdominal area. You have had pain and been nauseous for 3 days. Yesterday, you vomited twice. You have a fever; your temperature is 100 °F. You're not sure which department you should go to. Ask the nurse .

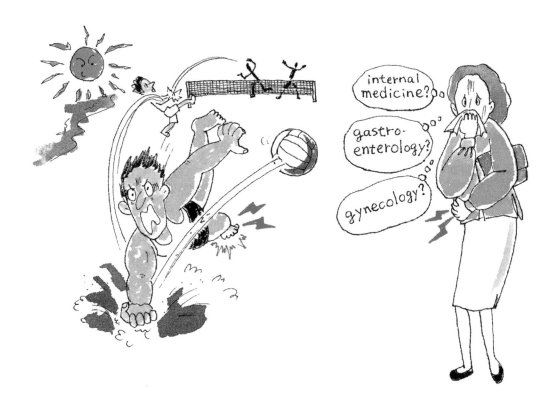

6 Activity Game : What's the sentence?

どうしましたか？

　このゲームは4人1組で行います. 先生がいろいろな症状の書かれたカードを渡します. カードをよく混ぜてから重ね, 机の上にふせてください. まず誰から始めるかを決め, 後は時計回りに行います. 最初の人は一番上のカードを引き, そこに書いてある症状を表す語を読んでください. するとその隣の人がそれを文章にして言います. たとえば "nausea" の場合, "I feel nauseous." "I am nauseous." "I am suffering from nausea." のように答えます.

nausea	例) "I feel nauseous." "I am nauseous." "I am suffering from nausea."

　正しい文章が言えたらカードがもらえます. その人が言えなかったら別の人が答えます. カードは正しく言えた人のものになります. 誰も答えられない場合は読み手がカードに書いてある答えを教え, そのカードは机の上に重ねてあるカードの中にもう一度混ぜてください. 終わった時に一番多くカードを持っている人の勝ちです.

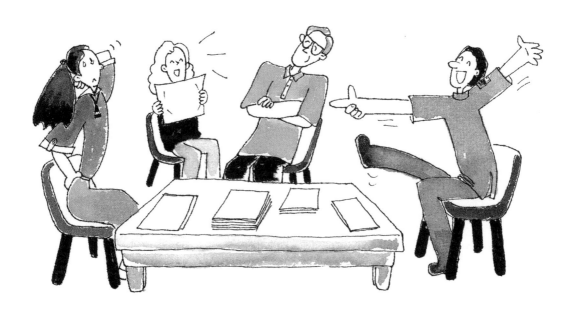

3 This is the nurses' station.

1 Activity Listening Practice

Audio 8

Listen to the conversations and choose the correct answers.

1. What time are visiting hours on Sunday ?
   a) from 2 to 7 pm   b) from 12 o'clock   c) from 11 to 7

2. On which days can women use the bath ?
   a) Saturday, Sunday, Monday
   b) Monday, Wednesday, Friday
   c) Tuesday, Thursday, Saturday

3. Where should patients who can walk eat their meals ?
   a) restaurant   b) their own room   c) dining room

4. What are the 3 places where we can find a nurse call button ?
   a) dining room, patient's bed, nurses' station
   b) bath, nurses' station, toilet
   c) toilet, bath, patient's bed

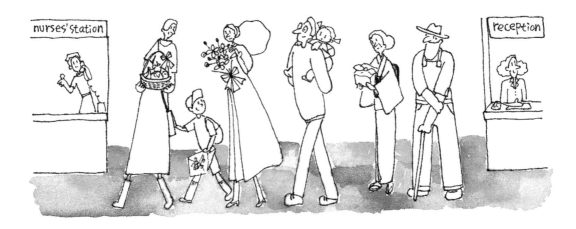

2 Activity **Checkpoint**

場所や備品を説明する

1. これはナースコールボタン(食堂)です.
This is the *nurse call button* (dining room).

2. ナースステーション(お手洗い, 浴室, 洗髪室, 相談室)はここです.
Here is the *nurses' station* (toilet, bath, shampoo room, consultation room).

3. 公衆電話(エレベーター)はここです.
Here are the *public telephones* (elevators).

4. 浴室は洗髪室の向かいです.
The *bath* is across from the *shampoo room*.

5. ナースステーションは診察室の隣です.
The *nurses' station* is next to the *examination room*.

6. 相談室は左(右)側です.
The *consultation room* is on the *left* (right) side.

7. 廊下をまっすぐ行って左(右)側にあります.
It's straight down the *hall* (corridor) and on the *left* (right).

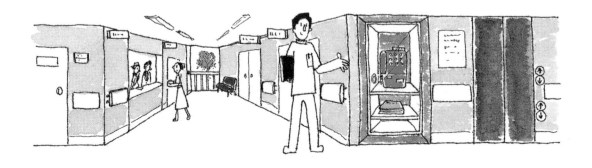

29

利用時間を説明する

1. 面会時間は午後 2 時から 7 時までです.
Visiting hours are from *2* to *7* pm.

2. 夕食は 5 時半です.
***Dinner* is served at *5:30*.**

3. 入浴は午後 1 時から 4 時の間です.
You can *take a bath*（use the bath）between *1* and *4* pm.

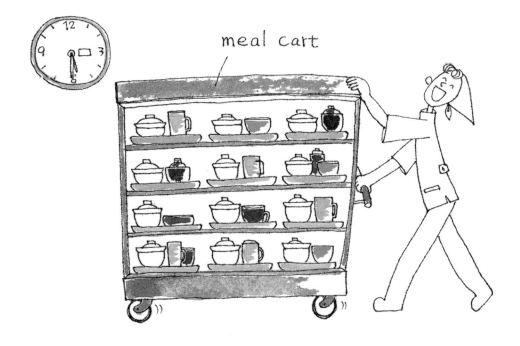

meal cart

3 Activity Dialog

Listen to the dialog and fill in the missing words.

■ **Admission Orientation**

    Masako : Hello Mr. Martin. I'm your 1) _____ , Masako Sato.
Mr. Martin : Hello.
    Masako : Your doctor is Dr. Kazuko Yamamoto. And the 2) _____
            is Yoshika Maeda.
Mr. Martin : I see.
    Masako : You can put your 3) _____ into this locker. Put your other
            possessions into the 4) _____ . This is the nurse call
            button. Please use this if you need a nurse's assistance. Please
            5) _____ after you put away your things.

■ **Later**

    Masako : Today I would like to give you an orientation 6) _____ .
            Please come with me.
Mr. Martin : OK.

31

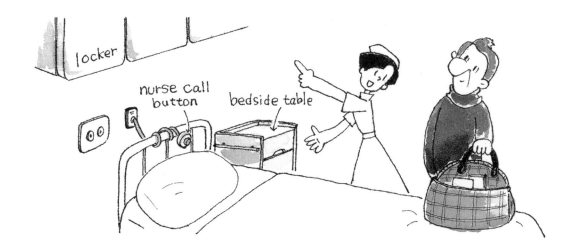

Masako : On your left is the 7) _____. If you receive a phone call, you can get your call here. 8) _____ the nurses' station is the consultation room.

Mr. Martin : Where can I make a phone call ?

Masako : There are pay phones 9) _____ outside this ward. 10) _____ on your left. If you need to have a urine test, please put the cup in this window. On your right is the sink where you can 11) _____ and brush your teeth.

Mr. Martin : 12) _____ ?

Masako : You can do your laundry here. There's a coin washing machine and dryer . You can use them 13) _____. The dining room is 14) _____.

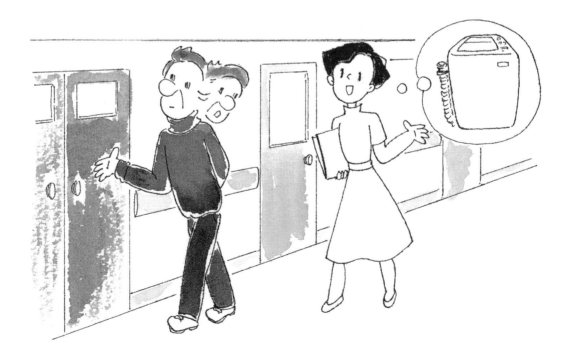

Activity

4 Puzzle 1 : Where is it ?

何の部屋でしょう？

下のヒントを読み，A, B, C, D, E がそれぞれ何の部屋か答えましょう（文中の left, right はこの地図上の位置です）．

・The <u>dining room</u> is across from Room 302.
・The <u>examination room</u> is next to the nurses' station, on the left.
・The <u>bath</u> is to the left of the toilets.
・The <u>laundry</u> is across from the nurses' station.
・The <u>consultation room</u> is to the right of the nurses' station.

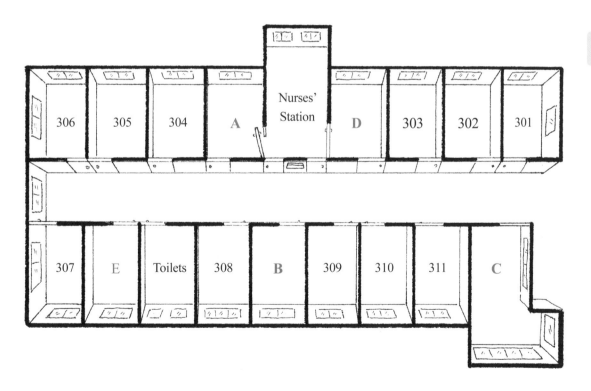

4 Puzzle 2 : What is it ?

Activity

どこにあるでしょう？

病院の中にはいろいろな備品があります。下のリストのものを絵の中から探して，番号をかっこ内に書きましょう。

Objects Used in a Hospital

( ) baby bottle	( ) IV drip	( ) stethoscope
( ) bedpan	( ) latex gloves	( ) stretcher
( ) blood pressure gauge	( ) medical chart	( ) syringe (needle)
( ) cast	( ) microscope	( ) thermometer
( ) crutches	( ) nurse call button	( ) vital signs monitor
( ) diaper	( ) oxygen	( ) walker
( ) emesis (kidney) basin	( ) scale	( ) X-ray
( ) examination table	( ) sling	
( ) gauze	( ) spouted water cup	

34

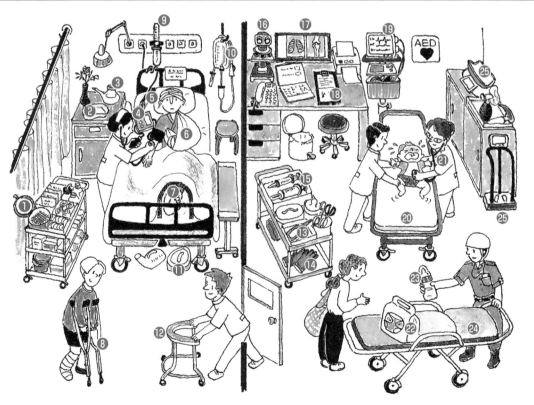

5 Role Play

病棟案内

　2人1組になり，患者役（A）と看護師役（B）を決め，カードの指示に従って病棟案内をしましょう．看護師は患者に，赤字で書かれた部分の説明をしてください．終わったら今度は役割を交替し，患者役（A）と看護師役（C）のカードを使って練習します．

Role Card A - Patient

Listen to the nurse's explanation. Ask questions. Fill in the missing information.

Your nurse: _____   *Head Nurse:* _____

Doctor: _____

Visiting Hours: _____

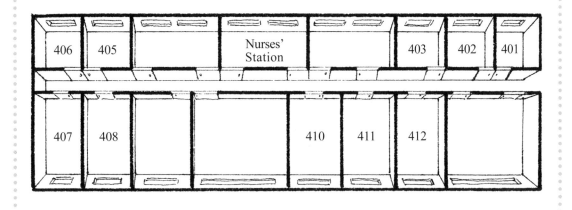

Role Card B - Nurse

Introduce yourself and tell the patient the information in red.

Nurse: (your name)   *Head Nurse: Masataka Fujino*

Doctor: Hiroko Sawamura

Visiting Hours: 2 PM - 7 PM

406	405	Consultation Room	Nurses' Station	Examination Room	403	402	401
407	408	Toilets	Bath 1-3 PM Men Mon Wed Fri Women Tue Thu Sat	410	411	412	Dining Room Breakfast 7:30 AM Lunch 12 Noon Dinner 6 PM

Role Card C - Nurse

Introduce yourself and tell the patient the information in red.

Nurse: (your name)   *Head Nurse: Mayumi Tanaka*

Doctor: Keizo Miyamoto

Visiting Hours: 1 PM - 8 PM

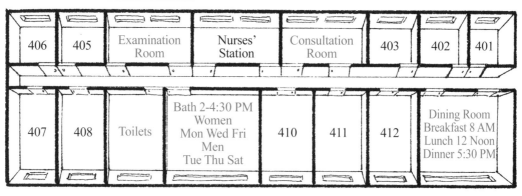

406	405	Examination Room	Nurses' Station	Consultation Room	403	402	401
407	408	Toilets	Bath 2-4:30 PM Women Mon Wed Fri Men Tue Thu Sat	410	411	412	Dining Room Breakfast 8 AM Lunch 12 Noon Dinner 5:30 PM

6 Activity Game : Bingo - What time is it ?

ビンゴゲーム 〜今何時？〜

　BINGO 1 のカードのマス目に，下の表から好きな時間を選んでばらばらに書き込みます．

　準備ができたらビンゴゲームを始めましょう．先生が表の中から 1 つずつ時間を読み上げていきます．あなたのビンゴカードにそれと同じ時間が書いてあれば，そのマス目を×印で消します．タテ・ヨコ・ナナメのどれか 1 列を全部消すことができたら上がりです．大きな声で "BINGO !" と言いましょう．

　次に BINGO 2 のカードを使って，もう一度ゲームを行います．

8:41	2:50	5:15	10:00	11:55	6:07	1:30	12:19
6:11	12:40	4:10	7:13	9:57	1:50	11:35	2:45
12:20	6:43	9:02	12:45	7:15	2:00	5:38	3:12
7:30	1:15	3:05	3:20	5:50	6:12	2:22	4:02
8:19	10:36	7:26	11:00	12:12	4:14	5:45	1:33

BINGO 1

		FREE		

BINGO 2

		FREE		

4 Are you suffering from any illnesses ?

1 Listening Practice

Listen to the conversations and choose the correct answers.

1. Who is Masayoshi Kitano ?
   a) He is Ms. Cane's doctor.   b) He is Ms. Cane's son.
   c) He is Ms. Cane's husband.

2. What restrictions does Ms. Cane have in her diet ?
   a) She doesn't eat rice.   b) She doesn't eat very salty food.
   c) She doesn't eat pork.

3. Does Ms. Cane drink alcohol ?
   a) No. She quit 2 years ago.   b) She drinks a glass every day.
   c) She drinks 7 glasses a day.

4. How did Ms. Cane's father die ?
   a) He had a heart attack.   b) He had hypertension.
   c) He had diabetes.

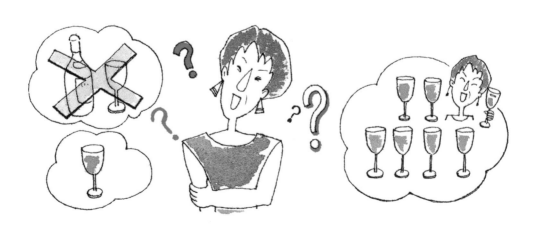

家族歴

1. 一番近いご親族はどなたですか.

Who is your next of kin ?

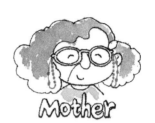

2. 緊急の際はどなたを呼びますか.

Who can we call in case of emergency ?

3. 家族構成を教えてください.

Please tell me your family composition.

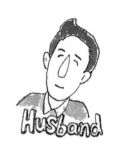

4. ご家族に病気の方はいますか.

Does anyone in your family suffer from a disease ?

いいえ. ／はい, 母は高血圧(症)です.

No. ／ Yes, my *mother* is suffering from *hypertension*.

5. その方は何で亡くなりましたか.

What did he *die* (pass away) from ?

肝硬変で亡くなりました.

He *died* (passed away) from *cirrhosis of the liver*.

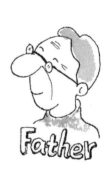

現病歴・既往歴

1. あなたには何か病気がありますか.

Do you suffer from any illness ?

いいえ, ありません. ／はい, 膵炎があります.

No, I don't. ／ Yes, I have *pancreatitis*.

2. この病気になってどのくらいになりますか.

How long have you had this illness ?
When did this illness start ?

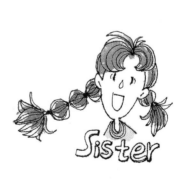

3. 何か大きな病気をしたことがありますか.

Have you ever had any serious illnesses?

> 前立腺癌になりました.
> **I had *prostate cancer*.**

4. それはいつでしたか.

When was that ?

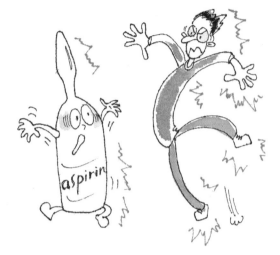

5. 何かアレルギーがありますか.

Do you have any allergies ?

> かびアレルギーがあります.
> **I'm allergic to *mold*.**

6. 何か薬に対するアレルギーがありますか.

Are you allergic to any medication ?

> はい, アスピリンアレルギーがあります.
> **Yes, I'm allergic to *aspirin*.**

食事・嗜好

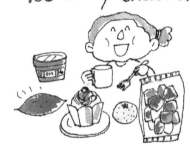

Too many snacks.

1. いつも食事はどんなものを食べていますか.

What is your usual diet ?

2. 何か食事の制限はありますか.

Do you have any restrictions in your diet ?

> 豚肉(肉, 脂肪の多い食べ物, 塩辛い食べ物)が食べられません.
> **I can't eat *pork*(meat, fatty food, salty food).**

3. 喫煙(飲酒)しますか. どれくらいの量(回数)ですか.

Do you *smoke*(drink)? How *much*(often)?

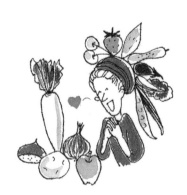

3 Dialog

Activity

Listen to the dialog and fill in the missing words.

■ Admission Interview

Masako : Is this the first time you've been admitted to a 1) _____ in Japan ?

Ms. Cane : Yes, it is.

Masako : What is the reason for your 2) _____ today ?

Ms. Cane : I have a pain in 3) _____ . My doctor said it's probably appendicitis.

Masako : Have you ever had any serious illnesses ?

Ms. Cane : I suffer from 4) _____ . I also have heart disease. And I was in a car accident 3 years ago, so I can't walk.

Masako : Are you 5) _____ any infectious diseases ?

Ms. Cane : No, I'm not.

Masako : 6) _____ had a blood transfusion ?

Ms. Cane : No, I haven't.

Masako : Are you taking any medication ?

Ms. Cane : Yes, 7) _____ medicine for my hypertension and heart disease.

Masako : Please give me your medication so I can show it to 8) _____.

Ms. Cane : OK.

41

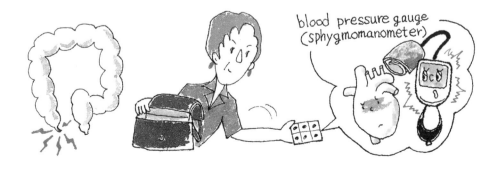

blood pressure gauge
(sphygmomanometer)

Masako : Do you have any 9)＿＿＿＿＿＿＿ ?

Ms. Cane : Yes, I'm allergic to peanuts.

Masako : Are you allergic to any medication ?

Ms. Cane : No, I'm not.

Masako : Do you need any help with your 10)＿＿＿＿＿＿＿＿＿ , for example with bathing or with your meals ?

Ms. Cane : Well, I use a wheelchair, so I need a little help, getting in and out of the 11)＿＿＿＿＿＿＿＿ . But I can usually bathe myself and I do the cooking in my house.

Masako : How is your eyesight and hearing ?

Ms. Cane : My 12)＿＿＿＿＿＿＿＿＿＿ are great.

Masako : How would you describe your 13)＿＿＿＿＿＿ ?

Ms. Cane : I think I'm cheerful and outgoing.

Masako : Could you tell me your religion ?

Ms. Cane : I'm Protestant.

Masako : Are you concerned or 14)＿＿＿＿＿＿＿＿ your illness or admission ?

Ms. Cane : I'm concerned about my surgery. And I'm worried that my nurses and doctor won't be able to speak English.

Masako : Please, don't worry. Your doctor 15)＿＿＿＿＿＿＿＿ . Some nurses can speak English, and you can ask for me if you need to talk about something.

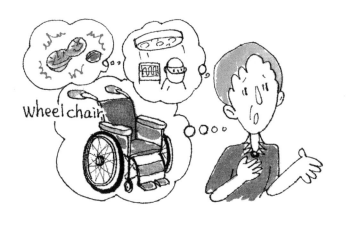

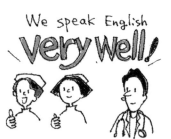

🔖 Heart Diseases

angina pectoris　狭心症

arrhythmia　不整脈

congestive heart failure

うっ血性心不全

myocardial infarction

心筋梗塞

🔖 Lung Diseases

(bronchial) asthma

（気管支）喘息

pleurisy (pleuritis)　胸膜炎

pneumonia　肺炎

pulmonary infarction　肺梗塞

🔖 Gastrointestinal Diseases

appendicitis　虫垂炎

duodenal ulcer　十二指腸潰瘍

gastric (stomach) ulcer

胃潰瘍

gastroenteritis　胃腸炎

hemorrhoid(s)　痔，痔疾

irritable bowel syndrome

過敏性腸症候群

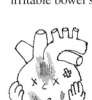

🔖 Liver, Gallbladder, Pancreas, Kidney Diseases

cirrhosis　肝硬変

gallstone(s)　胆石

hepatitis A (B, C)

A 型（B 型，C 型）肝炎

kidney stone(s)　腎結石

nephritis　腎炎

nephrotic syndrome

ネフローゼ症候群

pancreatitis　膵炎

🔖 Brain, Spinal, Nerve Diseases

Alzheimer's disease

アルツハイマー病

cerebral hemorrhage　脳出血

cerebral infarction　脳梗塞

epilepsy　てんかん

meningitis　髄膜炎

migraine (headache)

（片）頭痛

Parkinson's disease

パーキンソン病

stroke　（脳）卒中

🔖 Blood Diseases

anemia　貧血

hemophilia　血友病

leukemia　白血病

🔖 Infectious Diseases

AIDS (acquired immuno-
deficiency syndrome)

後天性免疫不全症候群, エイズ

cholera　コレラ

common cold　感冒，風邪

COVID-19 infection

新型コロナウイルス感染症

HIV (human immunodeficiency
virus)

ヒト免疫不全ウイルス

influenza (flu)

インフルエンザ，流行性感冒

malaria　マラリア

tuberculosis　結核

43

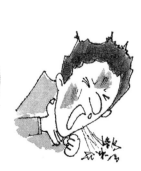

❤ Medical Terms : Diseases & Disorders

🖊 Skin Diseases

acne　にきび, 痤瘡（ざそう）

athlete's foot　足白癬, 水虫

eczema　湿疹

hives　じん麻疹

🖊 Skeletal, Muscular Diseases

fracture　骨折

herniated disc　椎間板ヘルニア

osteoporosis　骨粗鬆症（しょう）

🖊 Eye Diseases

cataract　白内障

glaucoma　緑内障

🖊 Ear, Nose, Throat Diseases

laryngitis　喉頭炎

Ménière's disease

　　　　　　　　メニエール病

(middle) ear infection　中耳炎

rhinitis　鼻炎

tonsillitis　扁桃炎

🖊 Other Diseases

alcoholism　アルコール依存症

allergy　アレルギー

anorexia (nervosa)

　　　　　　神経性食欲不振症

cystitis　膀胱炎

diabetes mellitus　糖尿病

gout　痛風

hypertension (high blood pressure)　高血圧（症）

hyperthyroidism

　　　　　　　甲状腺機能亢進症

hypothyroidism

　　　　　　　甲状腺機能低下症

rheumatoid arthritis

　　　　　　　　関節リウマチ

SLE (systemic lupus erythematosus)

　　　　　　全身性エリテマトーデス

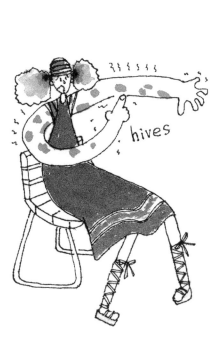

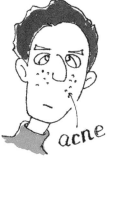

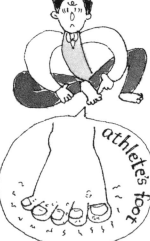

4 Puzzle : Diseases Word Search

潜伏している病気は？

下の図のタテ・ヨコ・ナナメに 18 の病名が隠れています．見つけ出して例のように丸で囲みましょう．

U	A	A	C	A	T	A	R	A	C	T	Q	R	E	A
W	X	S	P	L	E	U	K	E	M	I	A	S	M	F
H	L	E	T	P	K	S	S	N	A	A	A	E	F	X
S	A	P	T	H	E	A	E	D	B	E	Z	D	R	E
I	S	I	B	U	M	N	H	Y	S	C	B	U	A	E
S	I	L	R	B	O	A	D	I	E	Y	X	P	C	N
O	T	E	E	V	B	G	D	I	Q	X	V	A	T	O
L	I	P	D	A	L	T	A	V	C	R	M	J	U	T
U	L	S	E	H	R	I	J	M	D	I	B	M	R	S
C	L	Y	V	A	D	P	O	L	P	S	T	L	E	L
R	I	G	E	S	C	B	M	T	L	Z	E	I	Y	L
E	S	H	D	I	A	B	E	T	E	S	P	V	S	A
B	N	H	E	P	A	T	I	T	I	S	L	U	I	G
U	O	K	M	M	S	I	L	O	H	O	C	L	A	H
T	T	L	N	O	I	S	N	E	T	R	E	P	Y	H

45

Challenge! 英語の病名の下にそれぞれの日本語名を書きましょう．**Medical Terms** の病名リストを見ないでいくつできますか．

1. ASTHMA

2. AIDS

3. ALCOHOLISM

4. APPENDICITIS

5. CATARACT

6. DIABETES

7. ECZEMA

8. EPILEPSY

9. FRACTURE

10. GALLSTONE

11. GOUT

12. HEART DISEASE

13. HEPATITIS

14. HIVES

15. HYPERTENSION

16. LEUKEMIA

17. TONSILLITIS

18. TUBERCULOSIS

5 Role Play
Activity

病歴の聴取

　2人1組になり，看護師役（A）と患者（B）を決めてください．看護師は患者に質問して，入院時に患者の病歴などを記録するための書類（次頁）に記入しましょう．終わったら役割を交替し，患者役（C）と看護師役（A）のカードを使って練習します．

> **Role Card A - Nurse**
>
> *You are conducting an admission interview. Ask the patient about his/her family composition and family's medical history, patient's medical history, diet, dietary restrictions, smoking and drinking habits, religion and personality. Fill in the form.*

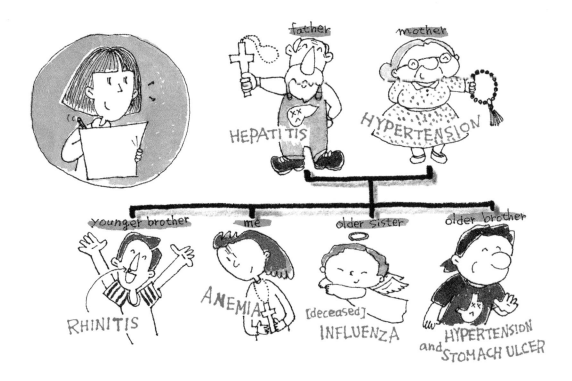

氏名 ＿＿＿＿＿＿＿＿＿＿＿＿＿　年齢 ＿＿＿＿＿　性別 ＿＿＿＿＿

1. 家族歴 （家族構成，家族病歴）

2. 患者病歴
　・既往歴　　　　　　　　　　　　　発病時期・期間

　・現病歴　　　　　　　　　　　　　発病時期・期間

　・アレルギーの有無

3. 生活歴
　・日常の食事

　・食事制限

　・飲酒・喫煙

4. 宗教

5. 性格

✐ Personality

anxious　不安な

calm　おだやかな，落ち着いた

cheerful　陽気な

depressed　憂うつな

friendly　好意的な，親切な

nervous　神経質な，臆病な

outgoing　社交的な，外向性の

quiet　静かな，控え目の

serious　まじめな

shy　はにかみ屋の，引っ込み思
　案の

optimist　楽天家，楽観論者

pessimist　厭世家，悲観論者

worrier (worrywart)

心配性の人

Role Card B - Patient ; Norma James, 39-year-old female

You are married. Your husband's name is Bob James. He is 43 years old. You have 2 children, an 8-year-old son, Rodney and a 12-year-old daughter, Mary. Your mother and father are alive. Your mother has been suffering from Alzheimer's disease for 2 years. Your father has been suffering from diabetes mellitus for 3 years. You have a younger brother who is healthy.

You have been suffering from asthma since you were 5 years old and had cervical cancer last year. You had a hysterectomy and are fine now. You are allergic to penicillin and peanuts.

You eat 3 meals a day. You don't eat pork and shellfish because you are Jewish. You don't smoke, but drink a glass of wine or beer almost every day.

Your personality is outgoing and cheerful.

Role Card C - Patient ; Steven Anderson, 53-year-old male

You live with your partner whose name Is Andrew Philips. He is 49 years old. Your mother is alive, but your father died 4 years ago from a stroke at the age of 79. He was suffering from heart disease for a long time. Your mother, who is 75, had her gallbladder removed 4 years ago. You have 2 younger sisters, Cynthia, who is 50 and Ellen, who is 48. Cynthia has gallbladder disease, but Ellen is healthy.

You have been suffering from hypertension since 2013. You have had a cough for 2 months. You are allergic to dust, mold and pollen.

You are a vegetarian; you don't eat any meat or fish. You don't smoke, but drink occasionally. You are Protestant.

Your personality is serious and you are nervous and a worrywart.

6 Activity　Game : Have you ever ?

こんな経験したことある？

　あなたのクラスメートがこれまでにどんな経験をしたか，次の質問を5人に尋ねてYES／NOを記入しましょう．　　例）"Have you ever been injured ?"

Have you ever	Name	Name	Name	Name	Name
been	injured ?	to China ?	to Hawaii ?	admitted to the HOSPITAL ?	to the U.S. ?
eaten	Mexican food ?	chocolate pudding ?	at a Buddhist temple ?	French food ?	snake ?
seen	Kabuki ?	Surgery ?	a traffic accident ?	a music concert ?	someone fall off a bicycle ?
	had stitches ?	had a fever of 40°C ?	had an injection ?	suffered from the flu ?	visited someone in the hospital ?

5 You need to have an MRI.

1 Activity Listening Practice

Audio 14

Listen to the conversations and choose the correct answers.

1. What is the nurse doing ?
   a) taking the patient's pulse   b) taking a blood sample
   c) doing a blood pressure test   d) doing an eye test

2. When should Mr. Silver have the tests done ?
   a) during his surgery   b) today   c) after his surgery
   d) after his admission

3. Which part of Ms. Jackson's body does the doctor want to examine ?
   a) her mouth   b) her stomach   c) her heart   d) her colon

4. What test does Mr. Kim need to have ?
   a) an RI   b) an X-ray   c) an EEG   d) an MRI

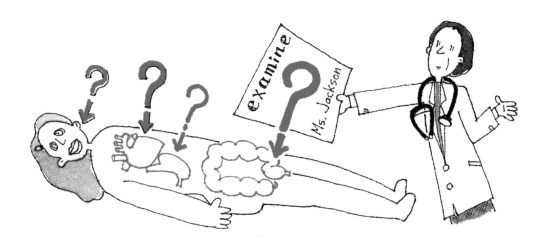

2 Activity **Checkpoint**

検査の指示をする

1. X線(脳波, 超音波, 大腸内視鏡)の検査が必要です.
You need to have an *X-ray*（EEG, echogram, colonoscopy）.

2. 洋服を脱いでこのガウンを着てください.
Please take off your *clothing*（clothes）and put on this gown.

3. この台に寝てください.
Please lie on this table.

4. 右を下にして(あおむけに, うつぶせに)寝てください.
Please lie on your *right side*（face up, face down）.

5. ここに立ってください.
Please stand here.

6. 動かないでください.
Please don't move.

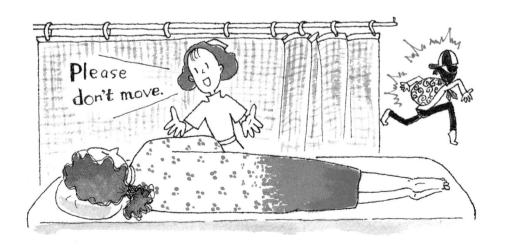

7. こぶしを握ってください.
Make a fist.

8. 息を吸って(吐いて)ください.
Inhale (**Exhale**).

9. 息を吸って(吐いて)そのまま止めてください.
Inhale (**Exhale**) **and hold your breath.**

10. 息を深く吸ってください.
Take a deep breath.

11. この薬(錠剤)を飲んでください.
Take *this medicine* (**these tablets**).

12. 熱を計ってください.
Take your temperature.

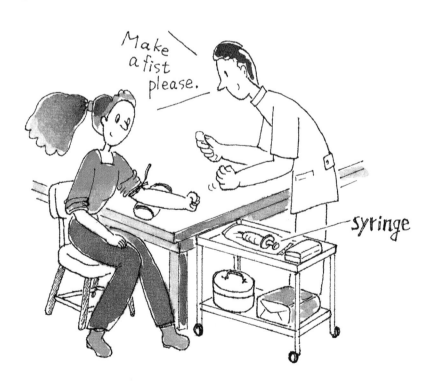

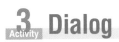

Listen to the dialog and fill in the missing words.

▪ Hospital Tests

Masako : Ms. Yang, you need to have 1) ＿＿＿＿＿＿＿ done this week.

Ms. Yang : What tests do I need ?

Masako : You need to have a chest 2) ＿＿＿＿＿, an EKG, a gastroscopy and an upper and a lower GI series.

Ms. Yang : I've had a 3) ＿＿＿＿＿＿ X-ray and an EKG before, but I never had a gastroscopy or GI series before. What kinds of tests are they ?

Masako : A gastroscopy and an upper GI series are to examine 4) ＿＿＿＿＿＿＿. In a gastroscopy, a doctor inserts a long tube through your mouth to your stomach.

Ms. Yang : Is it painful ?

Masako : No, it's 5) ＿＿＿＿＿ uncomfortable when you swallow the tube, but we'll give you some medicine to anesthetize your throat, so it won't 6) ＿＿＿＿＿ at all. Once the tube is in, the doctor can examine your esophagus, stomach and duodenum. It's best to relax during the test. If you want, we'll give you a sedative to help you relax.

Ms. Yang : I'm nervous 7) ＿＿＿＿＿＿ , so I think I'd like a sedative. What's a GI series ?

Masako : Well, an upper GI series is another test for your stomach and duodenum. In this test you drink some barium sulfate which coats your stomach so that the 8) ＿＿＿＿＿＿ of your stomach can be seen on an X-ray. Then the technician takes a lot of X-ray photographs. A lower GI series is a barium enema. In this case the barium is put into your colon by enema. The lining of your colon and rectum can be seen on X-rays.

53

Ms. Yang : Do I 9) _____ any other tests ?

Masako : Well, we'll check your blood and blood pressure every day and I'd like you to 10) _____ twice a day. After your doctor sees the results of your tests, she may decide to do some others.

■ **The Next Day**

Masako : You're going to have your lower GI series 11) _____. Today you can't have any solid food; we will give you a liquid meal for breakfast, lunch and dinner, such as broth and rice gruel. Please don't eat anything besides what you are served.

Ms. Yang : What is rice gruel ?

Masako : It's rice cooked with a lot of water for a long time until it's very soft.

Ms. Yang : I see. Do I need to take a laxative ?

Masako : Yes, you do. 12) _____ these 2 tablets at 9 pm and then please don't eat or drink anything after that.

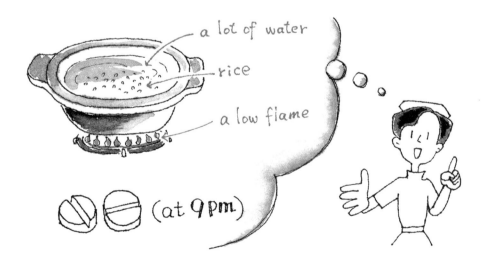

biopsy　生検, バイオプシー

blood pressure test　血圧測定

blood test　血液検査

bronchoscopy　気管支鏡検査

CAT (CT) scan (computerized axial tomography)
　　　　コンピュータ断層撮影

colonoscopy　大腸内視鏡検査

cystoscopy　膀胱鏡検査

ECG, EKG (electrocardio-gram, electrocardiography)
　　　　心電図, 心電図検査

EEG (electroencephalogram, electroencephalography)
　　　　脳波, 脳波検査

endoscopy　内視鏡検査

eye test　視力検査, 検眼

fecal occult blood test
　　　　便潜血検査

gastroscopy　胃内視鏡検査

hearing test　聴力検査

laparoscopy　腹腔鏡検査

lower GI series (barium enema)
　下部消化管造影(バリウム注腸)

lung function　肺機能検査

mammography
　乳房X線撮影, マンモグラフィ

MRI (magnetic resonance imaging)　磁気共鳴画像法

Pap test, Pap smear (uterine cancer screening)　パップ試験, パップスメア(子宮癌検査法)

rectal examination　直腸診

RI (radioisotope) scanning
　　　　ラジオアイソトープ検査

spinal tap (lumbar puncture)
　　　　腰椎穿刺

sputum test　喀痰検査

stool test　検便

thermography
　　　　サーモグラフィー

ultrasound (echogram, echo-graphy)　超音波, 超音波検査

upper GI series
　　　　上部消化管造影

urinalysis (urine test)
　　　　尿検査, 検尿

X-ray　X線, X線検査

55

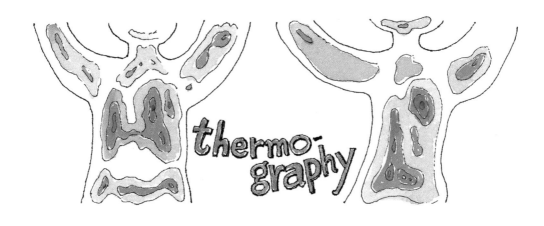

4 Activity Crossword Puzzle : Medical Tests

何の検査でしょう？

右ページのヒントを参考にして下の空欄を埋めましょう.

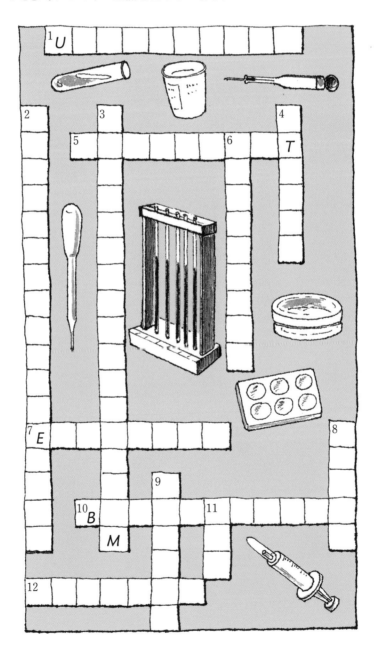

ACROSS

1 For this test, the patient puts a sample of urine into a cup which is then tested.

5 In this test, a sample of blood is taken from a person's vein.

7 Also called echography, echo or ultrasound, in this test, sound waves are passed into the body to find abnormalities.

10 In this test, a substance called barium sulfate is inserted by enema. Next, a lot of X-ray pictures of the colon and rectum are taken.

12 In this test, a doctor checks a person's vision.

DOWN

2 In this test, a blood pressure cuff is wrapped around the patient's upper arm to check his/her blood pressure.

3 Also called EKG, in this test, a doctor attaches electrodes to a person's chest, wrists and ankles to check the heart.

4 In this test, pictures of sections of the body can be made using computed tomography.

6 In this test, a doctor inserts a long thin tube into a person's body. The doctor can examine the inside of the body, take a photograph or take a tissue sample.

8 A test in which radiation is used to make a picture of the inside of the body, such as the bones.

9 In this test, a doctor removes a small piece of body tissue or some fluid to examine it for abnormalities under a microscope.

11 In this test, the patient is put into a long hollow machine and then magnetic waves are passed through the person's body. In this way a picture of the inside of a person's body can be made. This test is also called Magnetic Resonance Imaging.

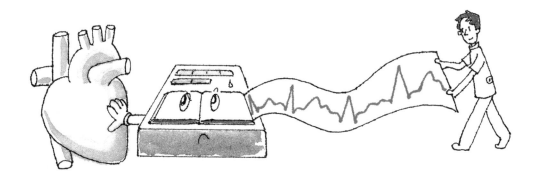

Activity **5** Role Play

検査の手順

　2人1組になり，看護師役(A)と患者役を決めてください．看護師役(A)の人はカードのとおりに英語で検査の手順を実演し，患者役の人はそれに従いましょう．下線部をヒントにしてください．終わったら役割を交替し，今度は看護師役(B)のカードを使って練習します．時間があればお互いにA，B両方の役をして，それぞれの検査を練習してみましょう．

Role Card A - Nurse；Taking a Blood Sample

　Read the instructions below several times until you understand; then act out the role play with your partner.

　You would like to take a blood sample from your patient. Prepare your syringe and vacuum tube. <u>Tell the patient to sit down and put her arm on the armrest.</u> <u>Tell your patient to make a fist.</u> *Tie a tourniquet around the patient's arm. Wipe the patient's arm with cotton soaked in alcohol. Remove the cover from the needle.* <u>Tell the patient, "It will sting a little."</u> *Insert the needle into the patient's vein. Push in the vacuum tube so the blood flows into the tube.* <u>Tell the patient to open her fist.</u> *Remove the tourniquet from the patient's arm. Place alcohol-soaked cotton over the puncture and remove the needle. Tape a band-aid on the puncture.* <u>Tell the patient to apply pressure for a few minutes.</u>

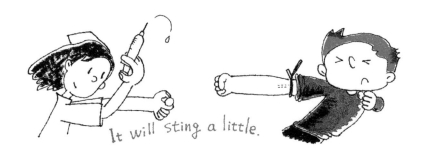

It will sting a little.

Role Card B - Nurse；Checking Respiration and Pulse

Read the instructions below several times until you understand; then act out the role play with your partner.

You would like to check your patient's respiration and pulse. Prepare your stethoscope. Tell your patient you would like to check his respiration and pulse. Ask your patient to sit up (down) and raise his shirt. Put the stethoscope against your patient's chest. Tell the patient to breathe (inhale) deeply and hold his breath. Tell the patient to exhale. Tell the patient to inhale and exhale several times as you listen to different spots. Next, tell the patient to turn around and put the stethoscope against the patient's back. Tell the patient to inhale and exhale several times as you listen to different spots. When you finish, tell the patient to pull down his shirt. Next, tell the patient you are going to take his pulse. Put your fingers against his wrist and time his pulse. When you are finished, tell the patient you are finished.

6 Game : Three Hints
Activity

検査名当てスリーヒントゲーム

これはグループ（できれば4人1組）で行うカルタゲームです．2組のカードのうち，Medical Tests Cards（答えのカード）は表を上にして机の上に広げておきます．Three Hints Cards（問題のカード）は各自に配り，それぞれ自分の前にふせておきます．

最初の人が手持ちのカードを1枚引き，そこに書いてある3つのヒントを1つずつ読み上げます．それ以外の人は答えのカードの中から，正しい検査名の書いてあるものを取ります．カードは取った人のものになります．今度は次の人が問題を読みます．このように順番に行い，最後に一番たくさんカードを持っている人の勝ちです．

6 You're going to have a baby!

1 Activity Listening Practice

Listen to the conversations and choose the correct answers.

1. What does the patient want ?
   a) She wants to have an abortion.
   b) She wants a pregnancy test.
   c) She wants a contraceptive.

2. How does Sarah know she's pregnant ?
   a) She missed her period.
   b) Her doctor gave her a pregnancy test.
   c) Her home pregnancy test was positive.

60

3. How old was the patient when she started menstruating ?
   a) She was 17 years old.   b) 2 weeks ago.
   c) She was 12 years old.

4. What kind of test does the patient want ?
   a) She wants a pregnancy test.   b) She wants an HIV test.
   c) She wants a herpes test.

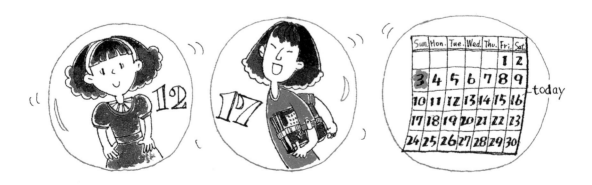

2 Checkpoint
Activity

産婦人科外来

1. 受診の目的は何ですか.

What's the purpose of your visit ?

妊娠(子宮癌)検査を受けたいのです.

I want a *pregnancy* (Pap) test.

HIV(梅毒, 淋病, ヘルペス)の検査を受けたいのです.

I want an *HIV* (syphilis, gonorrhea, herpes) test.

経口避妊薬(避妊リング)が欲しいのです.

I want *birth control pills* (an IUD).

ホルモン補充療法を受けたいのです.

I want hormone replacement therapy.

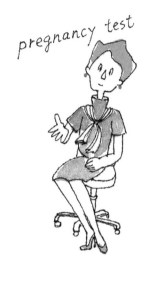
pregnancy test

2. 最終月経はいつでしたか.

When was your last period ?

3. 月経は順調ですか, 不順ですか.

Are your periods regular or irregular ?

4. 初潮はいつでしたか.

When did you start menstruating ?

61

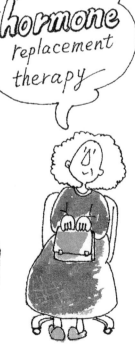
hormone replacement therapy

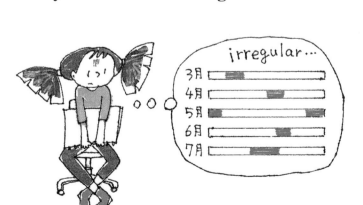
irregular...
3月
4月
5月
6月
7月

5. 受胎調節（避妊薬や避妊具，家族計画）はどうしていますか.

What kind of *birth control*（contraceptive, family planning）do you use？

コンドーム（避妊リング，経口避妊薬）を使っています.

I use *condoms*（an IUD, birth control pills）.

6. 今までに何回妊娠したことがありますか.

How many pregnancies have you had？

7. すべて生産^{せいさん}でしたか.

Have they all resulted in live births？

はい，そうです. ／いいえ，一度流産しました.

Yes, they have. ／ No, I had one miscarriage.

8. 死産したことがありますか.

Have you had any stillbirths？

9. 正常分娩でしたか，帝王切開でしたか.

Did you have a normal birth or a cesarean？

初産は正常で，2回目は帝王切開でした.

My first delivery was normal; the second was by cesarean section.

10. 流産や堕胎をしたことがありますか.

Have you had any miscarriages or abortions？

11. 閉経はいつでしたか. ／更年期はいつ始まりましたか.

When did you stop menstruating？ ／ When did you start menopause？

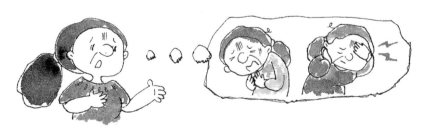

3 Dialog
Activity

Listen to the dialog and fill in the missing words.

■ **At the Maternity Clinic**

Mariko : Congratulations! I heard you're going 1) _____.

Mrs. Fisher : Thank you. The doctor said my expected date of delivery is September 7th.

Mariko : This booklet is a Maternal and Child Health Handbook. In Japanese, we say "Boshi Techo". 2) _____ _____ every time you visit. This will be a record of your pregnancy. And after your baby is born, it will be a record of your baby's health and inoculations.

Mrs. Fisher : What 3) _____ will the doctor do when I come for my check-ups ?

Mariko : She'll check your blood pressure, urine, and weight gain. She'll also do an internal examination and an echogram to check the development of the fetus.

■ **34 Weeks Later**

Mariko : How far apart are your contractions ?

Mrs. Fisher : 4) _____.

Mariko : Please change into your gown and we'll go to the 5) _____ room.

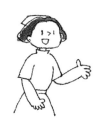

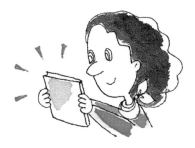

■ In the Labor Room

Mariko : You are fully dilated. 6) _____ the delivery room.

Dr. Taguchi : Your baby's head is crowning. Push, push. OK. Now, breathe. Breathe again. OK, now, push, 7) _____ , one more time. There you go. You have a beautiful baby girl.

Mariko : Let me clean her up and then you can hold her. Here you are.

■ After the Delivery - Mrs. Fisher's Room

Mariko : You can breast-feed your baby every time she cries. Please weigh her 8) _____ breast-feeding and write the weight here. After feeding her, please change her diaper.

Mrs. Fisher : I don't have too much milk yet and 9) _____ yellow.

Mariko : The first breast milk is called "colostrum". It's very 10) _____ .

■ Day of Discharge

Mariko : Your baby will 11) _____ of the time. But she may wake up frequently during the night for feeding. Be sure that you get enough rest.

Mrs. Fisher : When do I have to come back for a check-up ?

Mariko : Please come back in 4 weeks. But 12) _____ _____ like a fever, diarrhea, breathing difficulties, convulsions or jaundice, call the hospital immediately.

Mrs. Fisher : OK. Thank you very much for all your help.

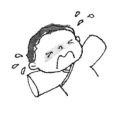 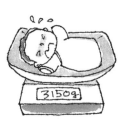 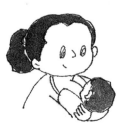 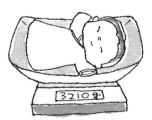

abortion　堕胎

afterbirth　後産

amniocentesis　羊水穿刺^{せん}

anesthesia　麻酔

Apgar score　アプガースコア

birth control　受胎調節

　birth control pills, the Pill

　　　　経口避妊薬，ピル

breech presentation

　　　骨盤位（逆子の胎位）

cell　細胞

cervix　子宮頸部

cervical cancer　子宮頸癌

cesarean section (delivery)

　　　　　　帝王切開

circumcision　包皮切断，割礼

colostrum　初乳

contraceptive　避妊薬，避妊具

contraction(s)　陣痛

convulsion(s)

　　　けいれん，ひきつけ

crowning　排臨

delivery　分娩

　delivery room　分娩室

development (of fetus)

　　　　（胎児の）発達

D & C (dilatation & curettage)

　　　拡張（子宮）掻爬^{そう は}

dilate

　　（特に身体の器官を）拡げる

eclampsia　子癇^{し かん}

effacement　子宮頸管展退度

embryo　胚，胎芽

emesis (vomiting)

　　　　　　嘔吐，つわり

epidural block　硬膜外ブロック

episiotomy　会陰切開術

expected date of delivery

　　　　　分娩予定日

face presentation

　　顔位（胎児顔面が先進する胎位）

fallopian tube　卵管

fetal monitoring

　　　　　胎児モニタリング

fetus　胎児

forceps　鉗子^{かん し}

genital chlamydial infection

　　　　　性器クラミジア感染症

gonorrhea　淋病

gynecologist　婦人科医

herpes　ヘルペス，疱疹

home pregnancy test

　　　　　　家庭用妊娠検査薬

hot flash

　（閉経期の）顔面紅潮，のぼせ

HRT (hormone replacement

　therapy)　ホルモン補充療法

intercourse　性交

　painful intercourse,

　intercourse pain　性交痛

65

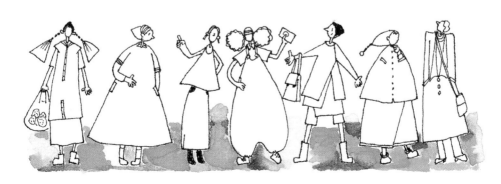

Medical Terms : Obstetrics & Gynecology

internal examination (exam)
　　　　　　　　　内診

IUD (intrauterine device)
　　　　　　　　避妊リング

jaundice　黄疸

labor　分娩, 陣痛

　　labor pain　陣痛

　　labor room　分娩室, 陣痛室

live birth　生児出生, 生産

maternity blues
　　　　　　マタニティブルー

menopause　閉経期, 更年期

menstruate　月経がある

　　menstrual pain　月経痛

midwife　助産師

miscarriage　流産

morning sickness
　　　　　早朝嘔吐, つわり

myoma of the uterus
　　　　　　　　子宮筋腫

neonate　新生児

normal birth　正常出産

normal delivery　正常分娩

obstetrician　産科医

organ　器官

ovulate　排卵する

Pap test, Pap smear
　　　パップ試験, パップスメア
　　　　　（子宮癌検査法）

period (monthly period)　月経

　　miss one's period　月経がない

placenta　胎盤

PMS (premenstrual syndrome)
　　　　　　　月経前症候群

postpartum blues
　　　　分娩後抑うつ（状態）

pre-eclampsia　子癇前症

pregnancy test　妊娠検査

premature delivery　早産

STD (sexually transmitted disease)
　　　　　　　性感染症

stillbirth　死産

syphilis　梅毒

trimester　3か月の期間
　　（妊娠期間の3分の1をさす）

ultrasound (echogram, echo-
　graphy)　超音波, 超音波検査

umbilical cord　へその緒, 臍帯

uterus (womb)　子宮

vacuum extraction　吸引分娩

vagina　腟

vaginal examination　腟内診

vaginitis　腟炎

weight gain　体重増加

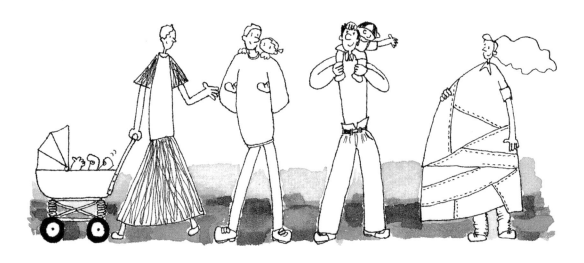

4 Activity Game : Your Childhood

どんな子どもだった？

クラスメート 3 人に幼児期の思い出について英語でインタビューしましょう．下の表に相手の名前と回答を記入してください．自分のグループ以外の人に聞くようにしましょう．

When you were a child ...	Name:	Name:	Name:
1. Did you have a "security blanket"? What was it ?			
2. What was your "comfort food" when you were sick?			
3. What was your special toy or book ?			
4. Did you go to nursery school or kindergarten ? From what age ?			
5. Did you have a pet? What was it ?			
6. Who was your special friend ?			
7. Did you have any serious injury ? What was it ?			
8. Were you ever hospital-ized?			

5 Activity **Role Play**

産婦人科予診票

2人1組になり，看護師役(A)と患者役(B)を決めてください．看護師役は患者役に質問して，下の予診票に記入しましょう．終わったら役割を交替し，今度は患者役(C)と看護師役(A)のカードを使って練習します．

Role Card A - Nurse

Your patient is a foreigner who can't understand Japanese. Ask your patient the questions to help her fill in the form.

氏名 _____ 年齢 _____

初潮年齢 _____

最終月経 _____

月経周期　　順調／不順 _____日型

閉経　　はい／いいえ　　閉経年齢 _____

妊娠回数 _____

分娩回数 _____

  1.　正常分娩／帝王切開

  2.　正常分娩／帝王切開

  3.　正常分娩／帝王切開

子どもの年齢・性別 _____

通常の避妊方法 _____

受診の目的 _____

主な症状 _____

いつから _____

その他の症状 _____

Role Card B - Patient ; Sylvia Franco, 55-year-old female

You started menstruating when you were 13 years old. Your periods are very irregular; your last period was 3 months ago. You have a period every few months.

You have 3 children, 2 sons, 24 and 26 years old and 1 daughter, 16 years old. You delivered your first 2 children by normal delivery and your daughter by cesarean section.

You use a condom as birth control.

You want to see the doctor about getting hormone replacement therapy. Your problem is that intercourse is painful. You've had this problem for about 3 years. Your other symptoms are hot flashes and cold sweats.

Role Card C - Patient ; Julia May Bookman, 24-year-old female

You had your first period when you were $11\frac{1}{2}$ years old. Your periods are regular, every 28 days. Your last period was 2 weeks ago.

You were pregnant once, but had a miscarriage in your 5th week. You don't have any children.

Now, you are using a condom as birth control, but you would like to change to the Pill. You want to see the doctor about getting the Pill.

You have no other problems or symptoms.

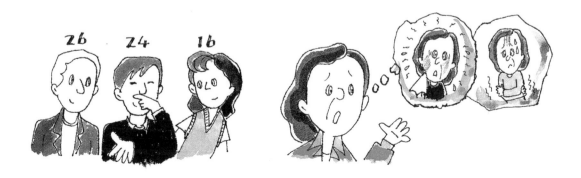

6 Crossword Puzzle : Having a baby!

赤ちゃんがやって来る

空欄には妊娠・出産に関する 18 の用語が入ります．右ページのヒントを読んで答えましょう．

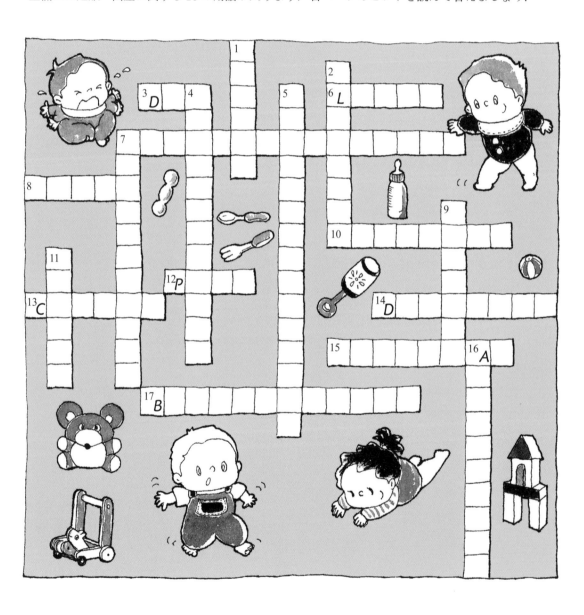

ACROSS

3 A procedure for doing an abortion by dilating the cervix and scraping the uterus.

6 The process of pushing out the fetus.

7 The feeling of nausea that many pregnant women experience in the early part of pregnancy.

8 The baby before it is born.

10 Artificial ending of a pregnancy.

12 Women take this as one form of birth control.

13 The lower end of the uterus, between the uterus and vagina.

14 Giving birth to a baby.

15 A test in which a doctor removes some cells from a woman's cervix to check them for cancer.

17 A way couples use to prevent becoming pregnant, such as a condom.

DOWN

1 A woman's sexual organ through which a baby is born in a normal delivery.

2 An organ lining the uterus, connected to the fetus by the umbilical cord and providing food for the fetus.

4 During birth, a woman experiences these. They help push out the fetus.

5 Delivery of a baby by cutting open the abdomen.

7 A spontaneous (happening by itself) ending of a pregnancy.

9 A nurse who is specially trained to deliver babies.

11 The part of a woman's body in which the fetus grows.

16 An assessment given to a newborn to check its physical condition.

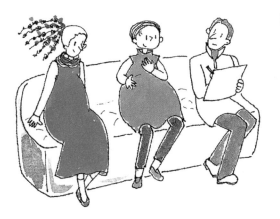
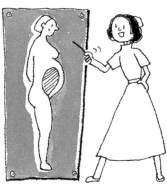

7 My baby has a fever.

1 Listening Practice
Activity

Audio 20

Listen to the conversations and choose the correct answers.

1. How long has Mary been sick ?
   a) 38.7℃   b) for 3 days   c) for 1 day

2. When did Howard have his first DPT inoculation ?
   a) three days ago   b) over a year ago   c) last week

3. What is the problem with Ms. Ryan's daughter ?
   a) She's vomiting.   b) She hit her head.   c) She's crying too much.

4. What vaccination does the father want for his son ?
   a) Diphtheria, pertussis, tetanus
   b) Japanese encephalitis
   c) Measles, mumps and rubella

72

　＊このユニットでは予防接種の内容が現在と異なるものがありますが，ここでは予防接種を英語で説
　　明する会話の一例としてご理解ください.

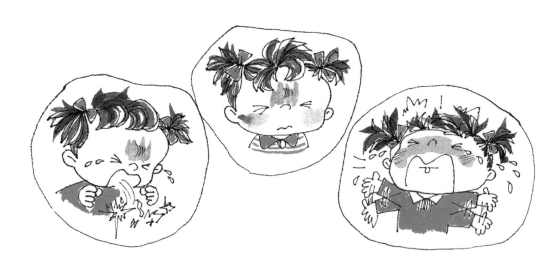

2 Checkpoint
Activity

予防接種の説明をする

1. 赤ちゃんにはどんな予防接種が必要ですか.

What *inoculations* (vaccinations, vaccine) should my baby get ?

DPT(ポリオ, 風疹, 麻疹, おたふくかぜ, 水疱瘡, BCG)の予防接種が必要です.

Your baby needs to get *DPT* (polio, rubella, measles, mumps, chickenpox, BCG) inoculation.

2. いつ接種すればいいですか.

When should *he* (she) get the inoculation ?

生後 2 か月から 1 歳の間です.

Between *2 months* and *1 year*.

生後 4 か月の時です.

At *4 months*.

73

3. 何回接種する必要がありますか.

How many times does *he* (she) need to have the inoculation ?

3 回(4 週間間隔で)接種する必要があります.

***He* (she) needs to get it *3 times* (at 4-week intervals).**

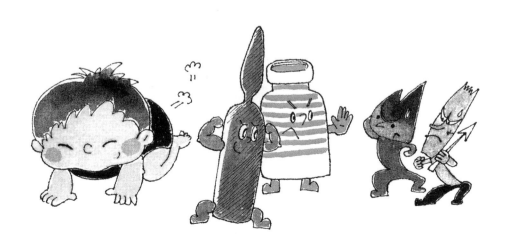

4. 追加接種が必要ですか.

Does my *son*（daughter）need to get a booster ?

はい，初回接種の 1 年後に追加接種が必要です.

Yes, *he*（she）needs a booster 1 year after the original inoculation.

4〜5 年ごとに追加接種が必要です.

***He*（She）needs a booster every 4 to 5 years.**

5. 予防接種はどこで受けられますか.

Where can my *son*（daughter）get the inoculations ?

いくつかの予防接種は保健所で受けられます.

***He*（She）can get some inoculations at the public health center.**

そのほかの予防接種は病院や診療所で受けられます.

Other inoculations are given at a hospital or a clinic.

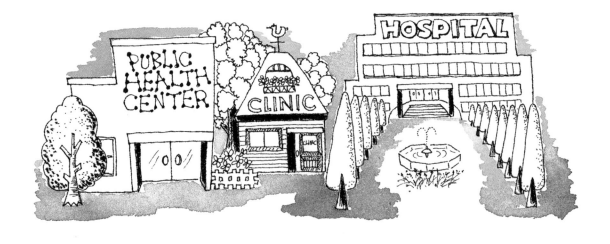

3. Activity Dialog

Listen to the dialog and fill in the missing words.

■ At the Pediatrician's

Akari : Joseph Sakata ?

Mrs. Sakata : Yes. 1) _____ Joseph.

Akari : How old is your son ?

Mrs. Sakata : He's 9 months old.

Akari : What seems 2) _____?

Mrs. Sakata : He's cranky and lethargic. He's been touching 3) _____ a lot.

Akari : Let's check his temperature. Please put this thermometer 4) _____ . Has he had any medical problems before ?

Mrs. Sakata : Well, he often seems to have a cold. He had roseola when he was about 3 months old.

Akari : Does Joseph 5) _____ , especially drug allergies ?

Mrs. Sakata : I don't think he's allergic to any drugs, but he's allergic to eggs.

Akari : OK. Let's see. He 6) _____ . His temperature is 38.5°C. Please wait; the doctor will see you soon.

75

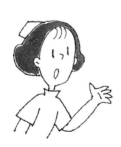

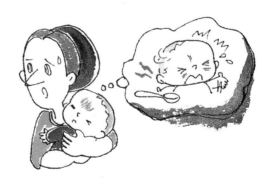

■ **Later**

Mrs. Sakata : The doctor said Joseph 7)_____ an ear infection. She said she'd give me some antibiotics and if the infection didn't clear up she said I'd better take Joseph to an ENT specialist.

Akari : Here's Joseph's medication. This is an antibiotic. It's a powder, so 8)_____ with some juice. Please give it to him three times a day after meals. And this yellow powder is for fever. Please give it to him if his temperature is higher than 38°C. 9)_____ or problems, please don't hesitate to call.

Mrs. Sakata : Thank you. Actually, I have some questions about Joseph's inoculations. He had DPT, Polio and BCG when he was about 5 months old. 10)_____ does he need ?

Akari : Well, he should have DPT 3 times, polio twice and BCG once.

Mrs. Sakata : I see. Are there any 11)_____ he needs ?

Akari : He should get rubella, measles, mumps and chickenpox vaccinations, but those are given after he is one year old. Then there's the inoculation for Japanese encephalitis.

Mrs. Sakata : 12)_____?

Akari : It's a disease carried by mosquitoes. Here, I can give you a schedule of inoculations in English.

Mrs. Sakata : Thank you.

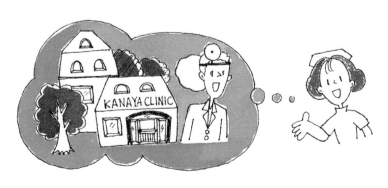

Type of Vaccination

BCG　BCG（結核予防ワクチン）

chickenpox　水疱瘡

DT (diphtheria / tetanus)
　　　　　ジフテリア，破傷風

DPT-IPV (diphtheria / pertussis /
　tetanus / polio)　ジフテリア，
　百日咳，破傷風，ポリオ

Japanese encephalitis
　　　　　　　　日本脳炎

hepatitis B　B型肝炎

Hib (haemophilus influenza
　type b)
　　ヒブ（インフルエンザ菌b型）

HPV (human papillomavirus)
　HPV（ヒトパピローマウイルス）

MMR (measles / mumps / rubella)
　　麻疹，おたふくかぜ，風疹

MR (measles / rubella)
　　　　　　　麻疹，風疹

mumps　おたふくかぜ

PCV (pneumococcal conjugate
　vaccine)　肺炎球菌ワクチン

rotavirus　ロタウイルス

live vaccine　生ワクチン

inactivated vaccine
　　　　　不活化ワクチン

Usage

stage 1　1期

booster　追加接種

interval　間隔

4 months or more after the
first shot　最初の接種後4か
月以上（間を空けて）

at 5-6 years old before enter-
ing elementary school
　　小学校入学前の5〜6歳で

between 6 and 24 weeks old
　　生後6〜24週の間で

77

＊最新の予防接種内容は国立感染症研究所ホームページなどをご確認ください.

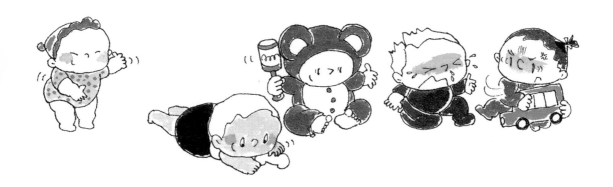

❤️ Medical Terms : Childhood Health Problems

🖊️ Diseases, Disorders

ADHD (attention deficit
hyperactivity disorder)
　　　　　注意欠如・多動症

atopic dermatitis
　　　　　アトピー性皮膚炎

autism　自閉症

bronchitis　気管支炎

colic　けいれん性腹痛, コリック

convulsion(s)
　　　　　けいれん, ひきつけ

croup　クループ, 偽膜性喉頭炎

Down's syndrome
　　　　　ダウン症候群

ear infection (otitis media)
　　　　　　　　中耳炎

food poisoning　食中毒

gastroenteritis　胃腸炎

hydrocephalus　水頭症

impetigo　膿痂疹, とびひ

Kawasaki disease (MCLS,
mucocutaneous lymph node
syndrome)　川崎病

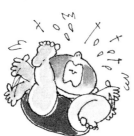

mental retardation
　　　　　精神発達遅滞

pinworm　蟯虫

rheumatic fever　リウマチ熱

roseola (-infantum)
　　　　　突発性発疹

SIDS (sudden infant death syndrome, crib death)
　　　　　乳幼児突然死症候群

stomatitis　口内炎

strep throat
　　　　(連鎖球菌性)咽頭炎

stuttering　吃音症

tonsillitis　扁桃炎

tuberculosis　結核

🖊️ Symptoms, Problems

bed-wetting　夜尿症

breathing difficulty　呼吸困難

child abuse　児童虐待, 幼児虐待

choking　窒息

crankiness　気難しさ, 機嫌悪さ

crying　啼泣, 泣くこと

cyanosis　チアノーゼ

dehydration　脱水

diaper rash　おむつかぶれ

edema　浮腫, むくみ

feeding problems　栄養の問題

heat rash　あせも, 汗疹

irritability　過敏性, 興奮性

lethargy　傾眠, 無気力

lice <louse　しらみ

sleeping problems　睡眠の問題

swallow foreign object
　　　　　誤飲する

teething
　　歯牙萌出, 歯が生えること

wheezing　喘鳴

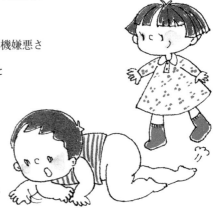

何の予防接種をしますか

次の単語を下の表の中から探して丸で囲んでください. 3～11 の英語の横に日本語名を書いてみましょう.

1. BCG
2. DPT
3. PERTUSSIS_____
4. RUBELLA_____
5. CHICKENPOX_____
6. MUMPS_____
7. POLIO_____
8. TETANUS_____
9. DIPHTHERIA_____
10. MEASLES_____

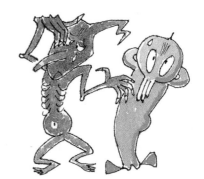

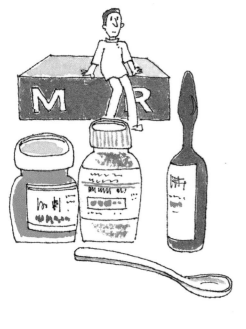

E	M	M	I	P	S	E	L	S	A	E	M
D	N	U	M	O	R	N	U	D	X	O	O
I	P	C	M	R	W	N	E	L	G	I	C
P	S	T	E	P	S	O	D	B	L	H	X
H	I	E	U	P	S	T	I	O	I	H	L
T	S	T	M	Z	H	F	P	C	X	X	F
H	S	A	J	D	O	A	K	O	A	X	X
E	U	N	G	Y	D	E	L	A	X	A	H
R	T	U	P	P	N	C	G	I	G	T	Q
I	R	S	T	P	N	L	J	I	T	C	U
A	E	G	O	F	A	D	W	J	D	I	B
J	P	X	V	A	L	L	E	B	U	R	S

Activity **5** Role Play

小児科外来

2人1組になり，看護師役(A)と小児患者の父親役(C) のカードを使って，ロールプレイをしながら小児科予診票に記入しましょう．次に役割を交替し，看護師役(B)と母親役(D)のカードを使ってロールプレイをしながら，予防接種申込書に記入しましょう．

Role Play Card A - Nurse

You are a nurse working in pediatrics. A girl, Susan, comes to your department with her father.

Ask her father questions to fill out the form below.

Tell the girl you will take a sample of her blood. Then tell the father and daughter the doctor will see her quickly.

小児科予診票

患者氏名 _____ 年齢 _____ 性別 _____

受診理由 _____

痛み　有／無　どのような痛み _____

痛みの部位 _____ いつから _____

他の症状 _____

既往歴

　病名 _____ 年齢 _____

　病名 _____ 年齢 _____

　病名 _____ 年齢 _____

　アレルギー _____

Role Play Card B - Nurse

You are a nurse working in pediatrics. A boy, Billy, comes to your department with his mother.

Ask his mother questions to fill out the form below.

Ms. Smith asks you what other inoculations he needs. Explain the inoculations he still needs.

Tell the mother, she must let the doctor know that Billy is allergic to eggs before he gets a measles vaccination.

Tell the mother, if Billy feels sick or has a high fever after the vaccination, she should bring him to the hospital.

予防接種申込書

患者氏名 _____ 年齢 _____ 性別 _____

希望する予防接種 _____

体温 _____

病歴　病名 _____ 年齢 _____

　　　病名 _____ 年齢 _____

　　　アレルギー _____

これまでの予防接種 _____ 年齢 _____

_____ _____

_____ _____

_____ _____

_____ _____

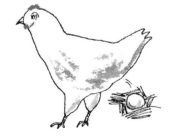
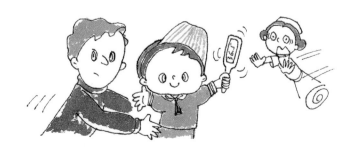

Role Card C - Patient's Father；Mr. Lee

You brought your 11-year-old daughter, Susan Lee, to the hospital because she is feeling sharp and severe pain in her right abdominal area. She's had pain for 2 days. She also feels nauseous and has a fever. Her temperature is 37.8 °C.

Susan had bronchial pneumonia when she was 5 years old. She's had asthma for about 3 years. She's allergic to penicillin, house dust and mold.

Role Card D - Patient's Mother；Ms. Smith

You brought your 2-year-old son, Billy Smith, to the hospital because you want him to get a chickenpox vaccination.

He is feeling fine. His temperature is 36.5 °C.

Billy had roseola when he was 6 months old. He often suffers from ear infections. The first time was when he was 1 year old.

Billy is allergic to eggs.

Billy had these inoculations:

MR - 1 time - at 1 year old

BCG - 1 time - at 9 months old

Ask the nurse what other inoculations he should get.

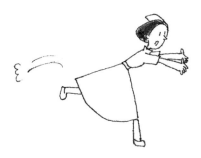
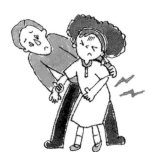

6 Game : Find Someone Who

あなたの過去を教えて

　教室内を自由に歩き回ってクラスメートに英語で質問し，子どもの頃に次のような経験をした人を見つけてください．該当者の名前を記入し，さらに関連する質問をあなたが考えて尋ねましょう．同じ相手にできる質問は3つまでです．早く全部の項目を埋めた人の勝ちです．

例）"Did you fly in an airplane ?" "Yes." "Where did you go ?" "I went to Hawaii."

When you were a child...

1. Could you play a musical instrument ?

Name _____

Q _____

A _____

2. Did you fly in an airplane ?

Name _____

Q _____

A _____

3. Did you live with your grandmother or grandfather ?

Name _____

Q _____

A _____

4. Could you ride a unicycle ?

Name _____

Q _____

A _____

5. Did you go to camp ?

Name _____

Q _____

A _____

6. Did you study English ?

Name _____

Q _____

A _____

7. Did you move several times ?

Name _____

Q _____

A _____

8. Could you swim ?

Name _____

Q _____

A _____

9. Did you go to an amusement park ?

Name _____

Q _____

A _____

10. Did you believe in Santa Claus ?

Name _____

Q _____

A _____

8 Your surgery will be tomorrow at 10 am.

1 Activity Listening Practice

Audio 23

Listen to the conversations and choose the correct answers.

1. How long does Mr. Edwards have to stay in the hospital after his surgery ?
   a) one week   b) three weeks   c) two weeks

2. What kind of surgery does Ms. Smith need ?
   a) pancreas surgery   b) hernia surgery   c) gallbladder surgery

3. What kind of anesthesia will they use for Mr. Horowitz' operation ?
   a) general anesthesia   b) local anesthesia   c) epidural anesthesia

4. Where can Ms. Cotto buy the things she needs ?
   a) at a convenience store   b) at the hospital shop
   c) at a department store

84

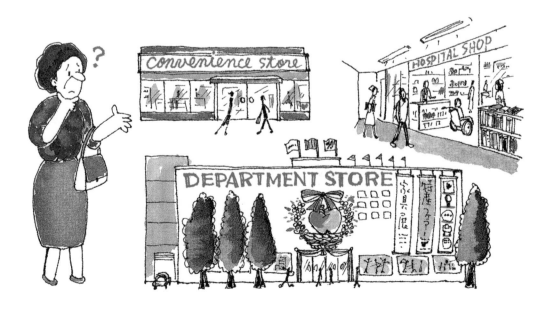

2 Checkpoint

Activity

手術の前に

1. 私にはどんな手術が必要ですか.

What kind of surgery do I need ?

腸の手術が必要です.

You need to have *intestinal* surgery.

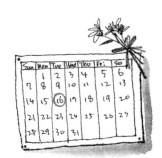

2. どんな麻酔を使うのですか.

What kind of anesthesia will they use ?

全身（局部, 硬膜外, 脊髄）麻酔を使います.

They'll use *general*（local, epidural, spinal）anesthesia.

3. 私の手術はいつですか.

When is my surgery ?

手術は火曜の午後になります.

Your surgery will be on *Tuesday* in the *afternoon*.

4. 手術が心配です.

I'm worried about my surgery.

心配いりませんよ. あなたの手術はとても簡単なものです.

Don't worry. Your surgery is quite simple.

担当の先生はベテランですよ.

Your doctor is an expert.

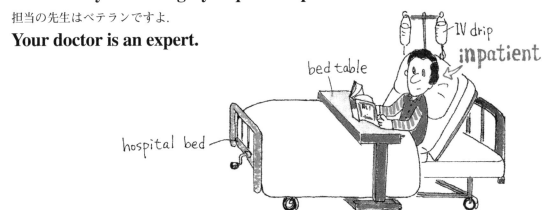

85

患者への説明

◇準備品

これが手術に必要な物のリストです.

Here is a list of things you need for your operation.

これらの品物は院内の売店で買えます.

You can get these items in the hospital shop.

◇医師の説明, 承諾書

医師が手術の説明をします.

Your doctor will explain your operation.

麻酔医が麻酔についてお話します.

Your anesthesiologist will talk to you about your anesthesia.

承諾書に署名する必要があります.

You have to sign a consent form.

◇手術前日

おなか(胸, 陰部)の毛を剃ります.

I have to shave your *abdomen* (chest, pubic area).

お風呂に入って洗髪してください.

Please take a bath and shampoo your hair.

食事は流動食になります.

You will have a liquid meal.

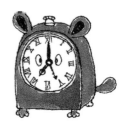

午後9時以降は何も飲食しないでください.

Don't eat or drink anything after *9 pm*.

この睡眠導入薬(下剤)を飲んでください.

Please take this *sleeping pill* (laxative).

午前5時に起きてください.

You have to wake up at *5 am*.

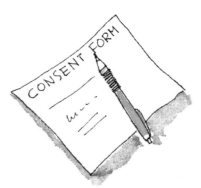

◇手術当日

入れ歯(メガネ，コンタクトレンズ，腕時計，装身具)をはずしてください．
Please remove your *dentures* (glasses, contacts, watch, jewelry).

お化粧はしないでください．
Don't use any make-up.

浣腸をします．できるだけ長く我慢してください．
I'm going to give you an enema; hold it in as long as possible.

膀胱にカテーテルを留置します．
I'm going to put a catheter in your bladder.

鼻から胃管を挿入します．
I'm going to insert a *stomach* (gastric) tube through your nose.

点滴を始めます．
I'm going to start your IV drip.

麻酔をかけます．
We're going to give you your anesthesia.

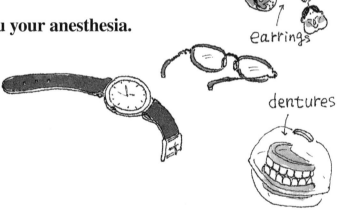

earrings

dentures

◇手術後

気管内チューブを抜きます．
We're going to remove your breathing tube.

病棟(病室，ICU，回復室)にお連れします．
We're going to bring you to *the ward* (your room, the ICU, the post-op room).

3 Activity **Dialog**

Listen to the dialog and fill in the missing words.

■ **Two Days Before Surgery**

Masako : Mr. Brown, your stomach surgery will be on 1) _____.
　　　　　There are some things you have to prepare for your surgery.

Mr. Brown : What do I need to prepare ?

Masako : You need to have 2 paper 2) _____, 2 bath towels, 3
　　　　　small towels, and your toothbrush and toothpaste. Besides
　　　　　that you have to have some special items for stomach surgery.

Mr. Brown : What special things do I need ?

Masako : Here is a list. You can get these things in the hospital shop.

Mr. Brown : OK. I'll go there now.

Masako : After you get them, 3) _____ on everything in water-
　　　　　proof ink and put it all in the shopping bags.

■ **The Day Before Surgery**

Masako : Today is going to be a busy day for you. This afternoon the
　　　　　anesthesiologist is going to explain about your anesthesia.
　　　　　Then later 4) _____ about your operation.

Mr. Brown : I see.

Masako : This morning, a nurse will shave your abdomen. And after that
　　　　　you should 5) _____ and shampoo your hair.

Mr. Brown : OK.

Masako : Dinner will be your last meal; it will be a liquid meal.
　　　　　6) _____ or plain tea until midnight.
　　　　　At 9 pm, I'd like you to take this sleeping pill.

■ The Day of Surgery - Before Surgery

Masako : It's time to wake up, Mr. Brown. 7) _____ ;
a nurse will give you an enema.

■ A Little Later

Masako : Mr. Brown, please 8) _____ , glasses and
dentures.   Please go to the bathroom, then change into this
surgical gown and rest in your bed.

Mr. Brown : I changed into my gown.

Masako : Good. I'm going to insert a catheter in your bladder. Then I'm
going to insert a stomach tube through your nose. Now, I'll
start your IV drip. Just rest in your bed until someone comes to
take you to the 9) _____ .

■ In the Operating Room

Anesthesiologist : Good morning Mr. Brown. After you're asleep we're
going to insert a breathing tube through your mouth. Now I
want to give you an epidural anesthesia. Please 10) _____
_____ and curve your spine as much as you can.

Mr. Brown : Like this ?

Anesthesiologist : Yes, that's good. OK, all done. Now lie on your back.

■ After Surgery - In the Recovery Room

Dr. Hamada : Mr. Brown, 11) _____ .
Everything went well. You're in the recovery room now. As
soon as the anesthesiologist says it's OK, we'll remove your
breathing tube and bring you back to the ward.

Medical Terms : Surgery

Types of Surgery

angioplasty　血管形成

appendectomy　虫垂切除

breast reconstruction　乳房再建

cholecystectomy　胆嚢切除

coronary artery bypass graft
　　　　　　　冠動脈バイパス術

embolectomy　塞栓摘出

gastrectomy　胃切除

heart-valve replacement
　　　　　　　心弁膜置換術

hemorrhoidectomy　痔核切除

hysterectomy　子宮摘出

lumpectomy　（乳房）腫瘤摘出

mastectomy　乳房切除

organ transplants (kidney, pan-
　　creas, heart, lung, liver, bone
　　marrow)　臓器移植（腎臓，
　　膵臓，心臓，肺，肝臓，骨髄）

plastic surgery　形成手術

pneumonectomy　肺切除

prostatectomy　前立腺切除

splenectomy　脾臓摘出

tonsillectomy　扁桃摘出

vasectomy　精管切除

Special Methods in Surgery

cryosurgery　凍結外科手術

laparoscopic surgery
　　　　　　　腹腔鏡手術

laser surgery　レーザー手術

Types of Anesthesia

epidural anesthesia　硬膜外麻酔

general anesthesia　全身麻酔

local (regional) anesthesia
　　　　　　　局部（局所）麻酔

sedative　鎮静剤

spinal anesthesia　脊椎麻酔

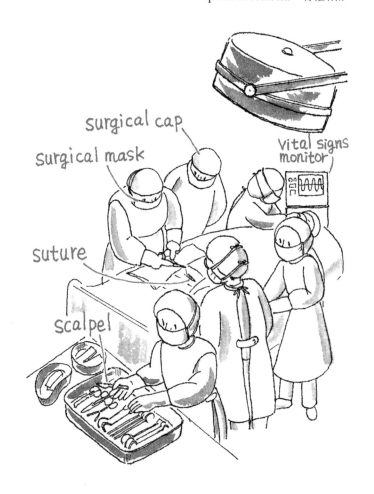

surgical cap

surgical mask

vital signs monitor

suture

scalpel

*手術の名称は「切断，外科手術」を意味する "-tomy" で終わるものが多いことに注目しましょう．

4 Puzzle : Body Parts
Activity

どこの部分でしょう？

下の表は人体内部のいろいろな器官のリストです．該当する番号を図の中から選んでかっこ内に書きましょう．

( ) appendix	( ) gallbladder	( ) ovary	( ) small intestine	( ) tonsil
( ) bladder	( ) heart	( ) pancreas	( ) spleen	( ) ureter
( ) bone	( ) kidney	( ) penis	( ) stomach	( ) uterus
( ) brain	( ) large intestine	( ) prostate	( ) testicle	( ) uvula
( ) duodenum	( ) liver	( ) rectum	( ) throat	( ) vagina
( ) esophagus	( ) lung	( ) rib	( ) thyroid	

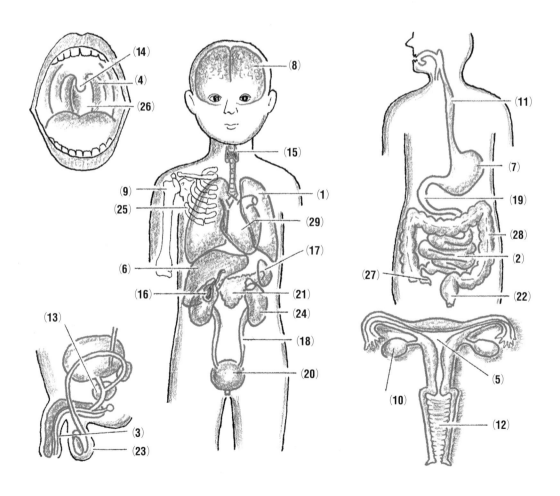

_{Activity} **5 Role Play**

手術の説明

　2人1組になり，看護師役(A)と患者役(C)を決めます．看護師役は患者役に詳しく手術の説明をしてください．単語だけではなくきちんと文章にして言いましょう．患者役から質問があればそれに答えてください．

　患者役は看護師役の説明を聞いて，カードの該当する答えに印をつけてください．看護師役の言うことがわからない時はどんどん質問しましょう．**Checkpoint** の表現や，Unit 1 の Emergency English を参考にしてください．

　終わったら役割を交替し，看護師役(B)と患者役(C)のカードを使って練習します．

> **Role Card A - Nurse**
>
> *Your patient is Barbara Jones. Explain about her surgery.*
>
> **Type of surgery:** *Mastectomy (removal of breast)*
>
> **Day/time of surgery:** *Thursday morning*
>
> **Type of anesthesia:** *Sedative, general*
>
> **Length of stay in the hospital:** *One week*
>
> **Items to prepare for surgery:** *2 bath towels, 3 small towels, a toothbrush and toothpaste, 2 paper shopping bags, 1 gown, 1 cotton T-binder, 1 pair of underpants, 1 spouted water cup, 2 chest binders, 1 pair of pajamas*
>
> **Day before surgery:** *Adhesive tape test. Abdomen, chest and armpit shaved. Take a bath; shampoo hair. Sign consent form. Last meal will be dinner, a regular meal. Take a sleeping pill.*
>
> **Morning of surgery:** *Enema at 6 am. Remove contacts, watch and jewelry. Don't wear make-up. Change into surgical gown and cap.*
> *Catheter and gastric tube will be inserted. Take a sedative.*

Role Card B - Nurse

Your patient's name is James Smith. Explain about his surgery.

Type of surgery: *Gastrectomy (stomach surgery)*

Day/time of surgery: *Tuesday afternoon*

Type of anesthesia: *Epidural, general*

Length of stay in the hospital: *3 weeks*

Items to prepare for surgery: *2 bath towels, 3 small towels, a toothbrush and toothpaste, 2 paper shopping bags, 2 gowns, 3 abdominal binders, 2 cotton T-binders, 1 pair of underpants, 2 spouted water cups*

Day before surgery: *Adhesive tape test. Chest and abdomen shaved. Take a bath. Sign consent form. Last meal will be dinner, a liquid meal.*

Morning of surgery: *Enema at 7 am. Remove glasses, watch and dentures. Change into surgical gown. Catheter and gastric tube will be inserted. IV drip will be started.*

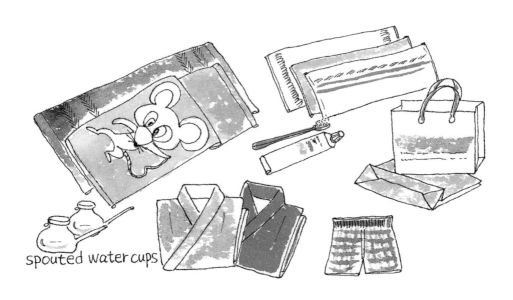

spouted water cups

Role Card C - Patient

Listen to the nurse's instructions and check what he/she says. Ask the nurse questions if you can't understand or hear something.

Type of surgery
[ ] *removal of gallbladder* [ ] *stomach surgery* [ ] *mastectomy*
[ ] *removal of pancreas* [ ] *intestinal surgery*

Day/time of surgery
• [ ] *Monday* [ ] *Tuesday* [ ] *Wednesday* [ ] *Thursday* [ ] *Friday*
• [ ] *morning* [ ] *afternoon*

Type of anesthesia
[ ] *sedative* [ ] *local* [ ] *epidural* [ ] *spinal* [ ] *general*

Length of stay in the hospital
• [ ] *one* [ ] *two* [ ] *three* [ ] *four* [ ] *five* [ ] *six*
• [ ] *day(s)* [ ] *week(s)* [ ] *month(s)*

Items to prepare for surgery
[ ] *towel* [ ] *toothpaste* [ ] *toothbrush* [ ] *shopping bag*
[ ] *gown* [ ] *abdominal binder* [ ] *T-binder* [ ] *chest binder*
[ ] *underpants* [ ] *pajamas* [ ] *spouted water cup*

Day before surgery
[ ] *adhesive tape test* [ ] *sign consent form* [ ] *take a bath*
[ ] *take a sleeping pill*
Shave [ ] *armpit* [ ] *abdomen* [ ] *chest* [ ] *pubic area*
     [ ] *neck area*
Last meal • [ ] *breakfast* [ ] *lunch* [ ] *dinner*
       • [ ] *regular* [ ] *liquid*

Morning of surgery
[ ] *enema* [ ] *bath* [ ] *change into surgical gown*
Remove [ ] *watch* [ ] *glasses* [ ] *contacts* [ ] *jewelry* [ ] *dentures*
Don't use [ ] *hair tonic* [ ] *make-up*
Items will be inserted [ ] *suppository* [ ] *gastric tube* [ ] *catheter*
               [ ] *IV drip*

Game : Pin the Organ on the Body

私のハートを返して

　これは福笑い形式のゲームです. まず大きな人体図(内部の器官がいくつか抜けているもの)を壁に貼ります. 誰か1人に心臓などの器官の絵カードを1つ渡し, 目隠しをしてぐるぐる回します. その人は自分で人体図のところまで行き, 器官の絵カードを図の正しい位置に貼らなくてはいけません. ほかの人たちは英語で次のような指示をして, 位置を教えてあげましょう.

例）Go forward. / Turn around. / Go *left* (right). / Turn *left* (right). /
　　Move your hand (a little) *up* (down, left, right).

　器官の絵をすべて貼り終わったらテキストにある人体図と比べ, どれだけ正確にできたか調べてみましょう.

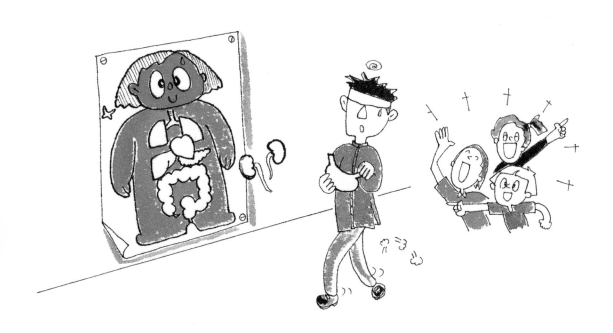

1 Listening Practice

Audio
27

Listen to the conversations and choose the correct answers.

1. What's Mr. Jones' problem ?
   a) He has a backache.   b) He has gas.   c) He is nauseous.
   d) He has a fever.

2. How much of her meals did Ms. Appleby eat yesterday ?
   a) She ate 30%.   b) She ate 50%.   c) She ate 75%.
   d) She ate 100%.

3. How many times did Maribel urinate ?
   a) 6 times   b) number one   c) 3 times   d) number two

4. How often should Ms. Silverstein take her medication ?
   a) 130 over 84   b) 3 times a day before meals
   c) 2 yellow tablets and 1 pink capsule
   d) 3 times a day after meals

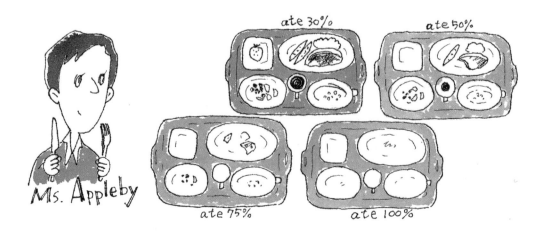

ate 30%   ate 50%

Ms. Appleby   ate 75%   ate 100%

2 Checkpoint

術後／日常看護

1. 気分(体調)はどうですか.

How are you feeling ?

2. 痛みはありますか.

Do you feel any pain ?

3. どこが痛みますか.

Where is the pain ?

背中が痛いです.

I have pain in my *back*.

手術したところがとても痛いです.

The *surgical site* is very painful.

4. どのくらい痛みますか.

How bad is the pain ?

ごく軽い(ややひどい, とても激しい)痛みです.

It's *very mild* (a little bad, very severe).

我慢できません.

I can't stand it.

5. 痛み止めの量を増やしましょう.

We'll increase your painkiller.

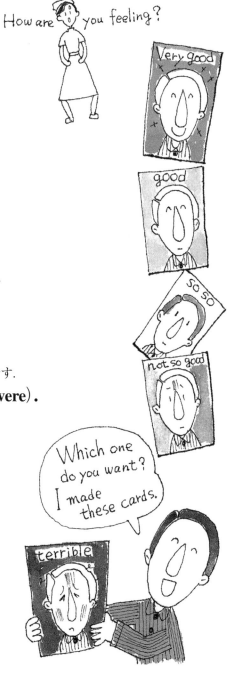

6. ぐあい悪いところがありますか.

Are you feeling any discomfort ?

> 頭痛がします.
>
> **I have** *a headache***.**
>
> 吐き気がします.
>
> **I feel** *nauseous***.**

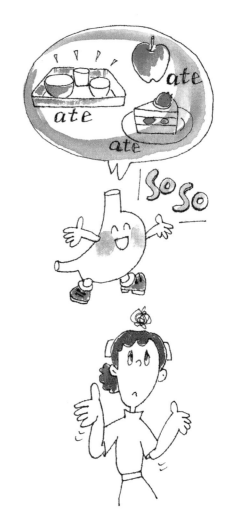

7. 食欲はありますか.

How is your appetite ?

8. 食事はどのくらい食べましたか.

How much of your meals did you eat ?

> 半分食べました.
>
> **I ate** $\frac{1}{2}$ (**50%**) **of my meals.**

9. 血圧を計らせてください.

Let me take your blood pressure.

> 血圧は上が 154,下が 85 です.

Your blood pressure is *154* **over** *85***.**

10. 注射をします.

I'm going to give you *a shot* (**an injection**)**.**

11. 抗菌薬(痛み止め)を投与しましょう.

I'm going to give you some *antibacterial agents* (**painkillers**)**.**

12. 昨日便通(排尿)は何回ありましたか.

How many times did you *move your bowels* (**urinate**) **yesterday ?**

> 1回(2回,6回)です.
>
> *Once* (**Twice, 6 times**)**.**

English-speaking people don't speak directly about urinating and having bowel movements. If they have to use the toilet, in America, they will ask, "Where's the restroom / bathroom / ladies' room / men's room / john?"   In England, they ask, "Where's the WC / loo?"

Young children may not know the words "urinate" and "bowel movement" and those who know them might feel embarrassed using them. Most commonly, "number one" is used for urination and "number two" is used for bowel movements. Adults might use ruder words like, "I have to pee / shit", but only among friends and certainly not in a hospital.

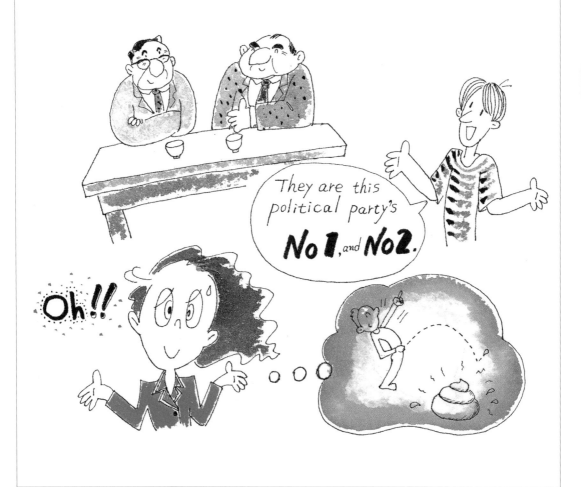

Activity **3** Dialog

Listen to the dialog and fill in the missing words.

■ **Post-Op ; In the Observation Room**

Ms. Roberts : 1) _____ ? Is my surgery over ?

    Masako : Your operation is over. You're in the observation room on your ward. You have to stay here until tomorrow. Are you feeling any pain ?

Ms. Roberts : Yes, my right side hurts.

    Masako : I'll give you a shot for the pain, but first I have to check 2) _____ and your blood pressure.

            OK. Here's a painkiller. Try to get some sleep.

■ **Later**

Ms. Roberts : I feel very thirsty. Can 3) _____ to drink ?

    Masako : Do you feel any nausea ?

Ms. Roberts : Yes, a little.

    Masako : Well, you can't drink anything yet, but you can 4) _____ _____. That will make you feel better.

Ms. Roberts : OK.

■ **Several Hours Later**

    Masako : How are you feeling ?

Ms. Roberts : I feel better, but 5) _____.

    Masako : Do you feel any nausea ?

Ms. Roberts : No, not at all.

emesis basin
(kidney)

■ The Next Morning

Masako : Good morning, Ms. Roberts. How are you this morning ?
Ms. Roberts : I'm 6) _____.
Masako : Your progress is going very well. 7) _____ remove your catheter and then you can be moved to your own room.

■ In Ms. Roberts Room

Ms. Roberts : Can I get out of bed today ?
Masako : Yes, the sooner you start moving, the sooner your wound will heal. But you 8) _____ the first time, so please ask a nurse to help you.
Ms. Roberts : I have to go to the bathroom.
Masako : OK. Please 9) _____ and put your feet over the side of your bed. Stand up slowly and hold onto my arm.

■ The Next Day

Masako : Everyone, please return 10) _____. The doctors are making their morning rounds.
Dr. Fujii : Nurse, please uncover Ms. Roberts' wound. Ms. Roberts, you are healing well. We can probably remove your stitches 11) _____.

■ Two Days Later

Masako : Good morning, Ms. Roberts. Here is 12) _____. Please take 2 capsules, 3 times a day after meals.

4 Activity Puzzle : Scrambled Words - Matching

何をしているところ？

ばらばらになった単語を並べ替えて正しい文を作りましょう．また，それぞれの文は右ページの A～
P のどの絵にあてはまるでしょうか． 1)～16) の番号を記入してください．

1) drip , finished , your , is _____ .

2) blood , I'm , take , going , sample , to , a _____ .

3) insert , into , going , I'm , suppository , anus , to , a , your

_____ .

4) change , surgical , into , please , gown , this

_____ .

5) temperature , please , your , take _____ .

6) is , your , pressure , 150 , blood , 85 , over _____ .

7) give , going , you , enema , I'm , an , to _____ .

8) need , bedpan , use , do , to , the , you _____ ?

9) an , to , I , injection , need , you , give _____ .

10) dressing , have , on , change , your , the , to , wound , I

_____ .

11) tomorrow , remove , the , will , doctor , stitches , your

_____ .

12) first , the , take , to , elevator , floor , the

_____ .

13) sample , cup , in , please , a urine , this , put

_____ .

14) listen , I , to , your , want , to , lungs _____ .

15) feel , do , nauseous , you _____ ?

16) call , toilet , a , to , need , please , if , you , the , to , go , nurse

_____ .

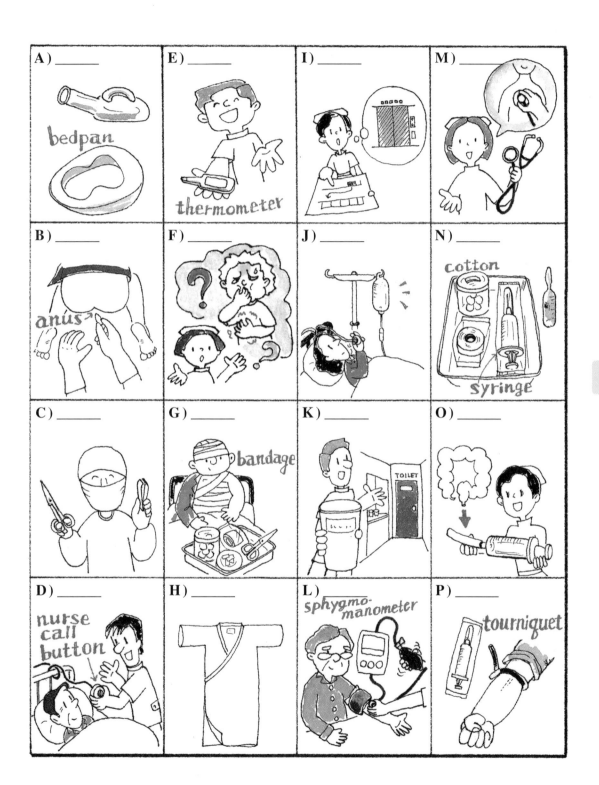

A) _____ bedpan

E) _____ thermometer

I) _____

M) _____

B) _____ anus

F) _____

J) _____

N) _____ cotton syringe

C) _____

G) _____ bandage

K) _____ TOILET

O) _____

D) _____ nurse call button

H) _____

L) _____ sphygmo- manometer

P) _____ tourniquet

❤ Medical Terms : Medicine

🔖 Internal Use Medicine

capsule　カプセル

liquid　水薬

pill　錠剤・丸薬

powder　粉薬

syrup　シロップ

tablet　錠剤

throat lozenge (troche)

トローチ

🔖 External Use Medicine

cream　クリーム

eye drops　点眼薬

inhalant　吸入薬

　cf.inhaler　吸入器(薬)

nose drops　点鼻薬

plaster　貼り薬

salve (ointment)　軟膏

spray　スプレー

suppository　坐薬

vaginal suppository　腟坐薬

🔖 How to Take Medicine

◇服用する

Take 3 yellow pills, 2 red and
white capsules, and 1 packet
of powder, 3 times a day
after meals.

Take this medication for 7
days.

◇挿入する

Insert the suppository in your
vagina (anus) every morning
and evening.

◇塗る

Spread the cream lightly on your
rash once a day.

◇使用する

Use the inhaler twice a day.

Take 4 puffs each time.

🔖 How Often to Take Medicine

once a day, twice a day,
3 times a day, 4 times a day

1 日 1 回, 2 回, 3 回, 4 回

every 4 hours　4 時間毎

after (before) every meal

毎食後(前)

after (before) *breakfast* (lunch,
dinner)

朝食(昼食, 夕食)後(前)

between meals　食間

before going to sleep　就寝前

when necessary　必要に応じて

as directed by your doctor

医師の指示どおりに

104

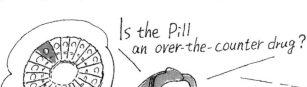

Is the Pill an over-the-counter drug?

No, it's a prescription drug.

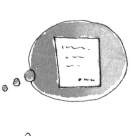

看護記録

　2人1組になり，看護師役(A)と患者役(C)を決めてください．看護師役は患者役に質問して，看護記録に記入しましょう．終わったら役割を交替し，今度は看護師役(B)と患者役(D)のカードを使って，同様に看護記録に記入します．

Role Card A - Nurse

Your patient is Jerry Lopez. He had gallbladder surgery.

Ask him how he is feeling, whether he has any pain, about his appetite, his bowel movements and urination, and his temperature.

Tell him you're going to take his blood pressure. It's 150 over 95. Give Mr. Lopez his medication. He should take the white tablet once a day before going to sleep.

Write the information on the Daily Report Chart on the next page.

Role Card B - Nurse

Your patient is Rosalie Galison. She had an abdominal hernia removed.

Ask her how she is feeling, whether she has any pain, about her appetite, her bowel movements and urination, and her temperature.

Tell her you're going to take a blood sample. Give Ms. Galison her medication. She should take 1 blue and white capsule 3 times a day after meals.

Write the information on the Daily Report Chart on the next page.

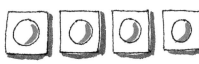

看護記録

患者名 _____

手術名 _____

主訴 _____

痛み　有／無　　部位 _____

食欲 _____

便通 _____ 回　　排尿 _____ 回

体温 _____　　血圧 _____

処方内容 _____

Role Card C - Patient

You are Jerry Lopez. You had gallbladder surgery. You're not feeling very well; you couldn't sleep last night because you felt nauseous. You have a pain in your lower back. Your appetite is not so good; you only ate about 30% of your meals yesterday. You had no bowel movements and urinated 7 times. Your temperature is 37.9˚.

Role Card D - Patient

You are Rosalie Galison. You had an abdominal hernia removed. You are feeling so-so. Your surgical site is very painful. Your appetite is so-so. You ate 60% of your meals. You had one bowel movement and urinated 6 times. Your temperature is 36.8˚.

6 Game : What's the object?

何をお探しですか？

　これはグループで行うカルタゲームです．カードは先生からもらってください．絵札は表を上にして机に広げ，読み札は重ねてふせておきます．誰か 1 人が読み手になり，一番上の読み札を取って，書いてある英単語を読みます．ほかの人はその単語を示す絵札を見つけましょう．（皆が順番に読み手になるようにしてください．）

　誰も絵札を取れない時は，書いてあった英単語を読み手が日本語で説明し，その読み札は元の束の中に戻して後で再挑戦します．一番多くカードを取った人の勝ちです．

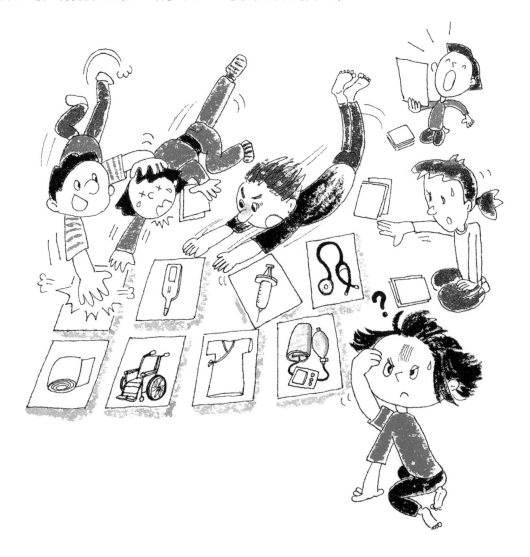

1 Listening Practice

Listen to the conversations and choose the correct answers.

1. What kind of foods can't Mrs. Lieberman eat ?
   a) She can't eat cheese or pork.
   b) She can't eat any meat.
   c) She can't eat shellfish and pork.
   d) She can't eat any meals.

2. Why is Billy worried ?
   a) He's worried because his stitches itch.
   b) He's worried because he's not healing well.
   c) He's worried because he's going to have an operation.
   d) He's worried it will hurt when the doctor takes out his stitches.

3. Why doesn't Mrs. Jennings want to have a blood transfusion ?
   a) Because she's afraid of getting HIV.
   b) Because she doesn't want surgery.
   c) Because of her religion.
   d) Because she's worried about her surgery.

4. What does Mr. Philips want ?
   a) He wants more painkillers.
   b) He wants to go home.
   c) He wants to talk to his doctor.
   d) He wants to stop taking morphine.

2 Activity Checkpoint

心のケア／文化や宗教の違い

1. 何か心配事や悩みがありますか.

Do you have any concerns or worries ?
Are you worried about anything ?

> ええ, 手術のことが心配です.
>
> **Yes, I'm worried about *my surgery*.**
>
> 本当に手術が必要なのでしょうか. 別の医師の意見も聞きたいのですが.
>
> **I don't know if I really need my surgery. I'd like to have a second opinion.**

2. ご心配なら一緒に主治医と話してみましょう.

If you are worried, let's talk with your doctor.

> 主治医にあなたの治療のことを話して(聞いて)みます.

I'll *talk to* (ask) your doctor about your treatment.

3. あなたの宗教は何ですか.

What's your religion ?
What religion are you ?

> 私はカトリック教徒(プロテスタント, イスラム教徒, ユダヤ教徒, 仏教徒, ヒンズー教徒, エホバの証人)です.
>
> **I'm *Catholic* (Protestant, Islamic, Jewish, Buddhist, Hindu, a Jehovah's Witness).**

4. 何か宗教上の制約がありますか.

Do you have any restrictions because of your religion ?

> 私は輸血が受けられません.
>
> **I can't have a blood transfusion.**

5. 何か食事制限がありますか.

Do you have any dietary restrictions ?

私は菜食主義です.

I'm a vegetarian.

豚肉 (牛肉) が食べられません.

I can't eat *pork*（beef）.

ユダヤ教の法にかなった (清浄な) ものしか食べられません.

I can only eat kosher food.

6. 何か宗教上の要望がありますか.

Do you have any requirements because of your religion ?

ユダヤ教徒なので男の子が生まれたら割礼をしなければなりません.

Well, I'm Jewish, so my baby has to be circumcised if it's a boy.

7. 薬草治療も含めて何か薬を飲んでいますか.

Are you taking any medications, including herbal medication ?

漢方薬を使っています.

I'm using Chinese medicine.

8. 服用中の薬があれば見せてください.

Please show me any medications you are using.

9. 個室がいいですか, 4 人部屋がいいですか.

Would you like a private room or a 4-person room ?

個室がいいです.

I'd like a private room.

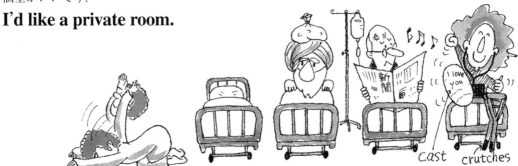

cast   crutches

3 Activity Dialog

Listen to the dialog and fill in the missing words.

■ A Nurse is Visiting from America

Masako : Hello, I'm Masako Sato. 1)_____.

Carol : How do you do ? My name is Carol Phillips.

Masako : Is this your 2)_____ to Japan ?

Carol : No, it isn't. I was an exchange student in Japan for a year in my university days.

■ Later

Masako : We sometimes have 3)_____. Is there anything we should be careful about when caring for them ?

Carol : In America, we have to treat patients of many different nationalities, religions and cultural backgrounds. The most important thing is for doctors and nurses to realize that 4)_____.

Masako : What are the most important differences ?

Carol : We have to be careful about different peoples' attitudes towards doctors, hospitals and healing. For example, some ethnic groups, such as Koreans and Chinese, use herbal medicines which may react adversely with the drugs the doctor prescribes.

Masako : What are some 5)_____American patients ?

Carol : I think 6)_____ between Japanese and Americans is that Americans want to know everything about their disease and treatment. They ask the doctor many questions.

Masako : Yes, I think that Japanese patients are more passive.

Carol : 7)_____ you have to consider is a person's religion. For example, if a person is Catholic they need to see a priest before

111

they die. Some religions don't permit blood transfusions. Then, some people have dietary restrictions. Islamic or Jewish people cannot eat pork. So it's important to find out about 8) _____ and ask if he or she has any restrictions or special needs.

Masako : I didn't realize that religion is so important. Well, I'm glad I talked with you. By the way, there's an Englishman on my ward. I think 9) _____ to talk with you.

■ On the Ward

Masako : Mr. Wilson, this is Carol Philips. She's a 10) _____ _____ America.

Mr. Wilson : How do you do ? I'm pleased to meet you.

Carol : How are you Mr. Wilson ? 11) _____ being in a Japanese hospital ?

Mr. Wilson : Well, I'm really glad because Ms. Sato and my doctor can speak English.

Carol : Do you have any worries or concerns ?

Mr. Wilson : To tell the truth, 12) _____ my surgery. I'm wondering whether I really need it. In the west, we always get a second opinion, but in Japan it's not the custom.

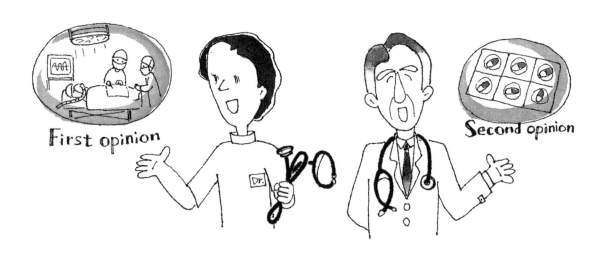

First opinion   Second opinion

Carol : Yes, I can understand your concern. Perhaps, you should talk to your doctor again. Would you like me to be there when you talk to your doctor ? Maybe 13)_____ anything you don't understand.

Mr. Wilson : Yes, I'd like you to be there. My doctor said he'd come by at 8 o'clock this evening.

Carol : I'll be sure to come here before 8.

Mr. Wilson : Well, Ms. Philips, I was glad to have 14)_____with you.

■ In the Nurses' Lounge

Masako : I'm really glad that you spoke with Mr. Wilson. I 15)_____ how worried he was.

Carol : I'm glad I was able to help.

Masako : I realize now that the best way is to ask the patient directly about his concerns or wishes.

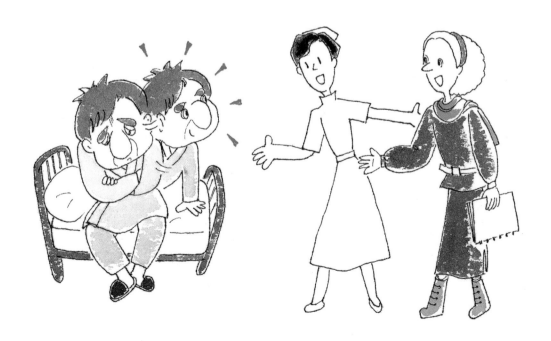

4 Activity Puzzle : Quiz

各国の文化や宗教

各国の文化や宗教についてどれくらい知っていますか. あなたの知識をチェックしてみましょう. ただし答えは1つとは限りません.

1. Which is the oldest religion ?
   a) Buddhism   b) Judaism   c) Hinduism

2. Which religion has the most followers ?
   a) Buddhism   b) Christianity   c) Muslim

3. Which groups of people use herbal medicine ?
   a) Chinese   b) Native Americans   c) Koreans

4. Which religion prohibits the eating of beef ?
   a) Judaism   b) Muslim   c) Hinduism

5. Which nationality believes that touching the head of a person may take away the person's spirit ?
   a) Vietnamese   b) Japanese   c) Polish

6. Which religion prohibits smoking tobacco and blood transfusions ?
   a) Shintoism   b) Jehovah's Witnesses   c) Judaism

7. Which religion prohibits abortion and divorce ?
   a) Judaism   b) Catholicism   c) Buddhism

8. Which religions forbid suicide ?
   a) Buddhist   b) Islam   c) Catholic

9. In which religion do boys become circumcised soon after birth ?
   a) Christianity   b) Buddhism   c) Judaism

10. In which religion do women have to have a female doctor or midwife to deliver their baby ?
    a) Buddhism   b) Judaism   c) Muslim

5 Role Play

心配事への対応

　2人1組になり，看護師役(A)と患者役(C)を決めてください．看護師役は患者役に質問して，入院患者面接票に記入しましょう．終わったら役割を交替し，今度は看護師役(B)と患者役(D)のカードを使って，同様に入院患者面接票に記入します．

Role Card A - Nurse

Ask your patient questions to fill out the form.

　Your patient is Muslim and can't eat pork.

　He is worried that the insulin he needs for his disease is made from a pig's pancreas.

　Tell him that you will explain his problem to his doctor and see if they can use insulin from sheep or oxen instead of pigs.

Role Card B - Nurse

Ask your patient questions to fill out the form.

　Your patient is very old and can't walk by herself.

　Tell your patient you will put a portable toilet next to her bed and a nurse will help her use the toilet.

　Your patient is worried whether she really needs to have the surgery. Tell her you'll ask her doctor if there is some other way to treat her ulcer.

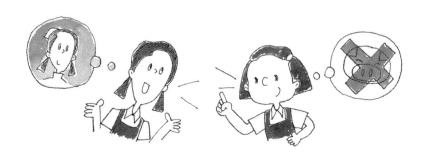

入院患者面接票

氏名＿＿＿＿＿＿＿＿＿＿＿＿＿ 年齢＿＿＿＿＿＿＿ 性別＿＿＿＿＿

入院理由＿＿＿＿＿＿＿＿＿＿＿＿＿＿＿＿＿ 部屋の希望

国籍＿＿＿＿＿＿＿＿＿ 宗教＿＿＿＿＿＿＿＿＿ 個室／４人部屋

宗教上の制約＿＿＿＿＿＿＿＿＿＿＿＿＿＿＿＿＿

要望・特記事項＿＿＿＿＿＿＿＿＿＿＿＿＿＿＿

服用中の薬＿＿＿＿＿＿＿＿＿＿＿＿＿＿＿＿＿

悩み・心配事

＿＿＿＿＿＿＿＿＿＿＿＿＿＿＿＿＿＿＿＿＿＿＿

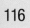

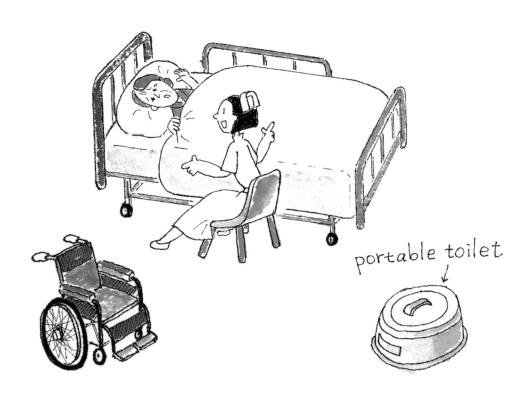

portable toilet

Role Card C - Patient ; Abdul Mohammed, 46-year-old male

You were admitted because you have diabetes mellitus.

You are Egyptian and your religion is Muslim. Your religion doesn't permit you to eat pork.

You'd like to stay in a 4-person room.

You are taking medication for hypertension.

You are worried because you must have insulin to treat your diabetes and you heard that insulin is made from the pancreas of a pig. You can't take any part from a pig into your body.

Role Card D - Patient ; Sun Wei Lin, 85-year-old female

You were admitted to have surgery for a gastric ulcer.

You are Chinese and your religion is Buddhist. You don't have any special restrictions because of your religion.

You can't walk by yourself, so you use a wheelchair.

You'd like to stay in a private room.

You are taking many kinds of Chinese medicine.

You are really scared of having surgery. You are very old, so you are wondering whether you should really have it.

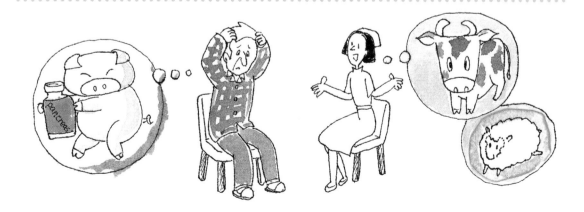

6 Game : What's the question?

Activity

何を聞かれたのでしょう？

　グループに分かれ，各自のコマ（消しゴムなど）を決めてゲームボードの START のところに置きます．付属のカードを先生からもらい，1枚ずつ切り離したらよく繰ってふせておきます．

　1人ずつ順番にさいころか硬貨を投げ，出た数だけコマを進めてください（硬貨の場合は表が出たら1，裏が出たら2進む）．コマが止まった箇所の英文を声に出して読み，指示に従って質問に答えます．

　TAKE A CARD と書いてあるところに止まった人は札を1枚取り，書いてある英文を声に出して読みます．ほかの人はその文が答えとなるような質問文を言わなければなりません．一番早くゴールした人の勝ちです．時間があれば全員がゴールするまで続けます．

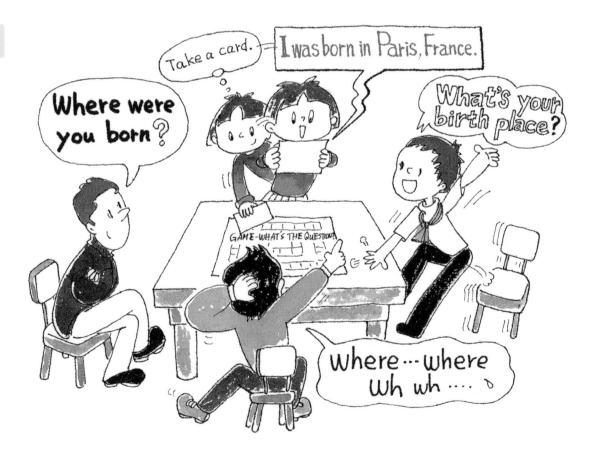

GAME-WHAT'S THE QUESTION?

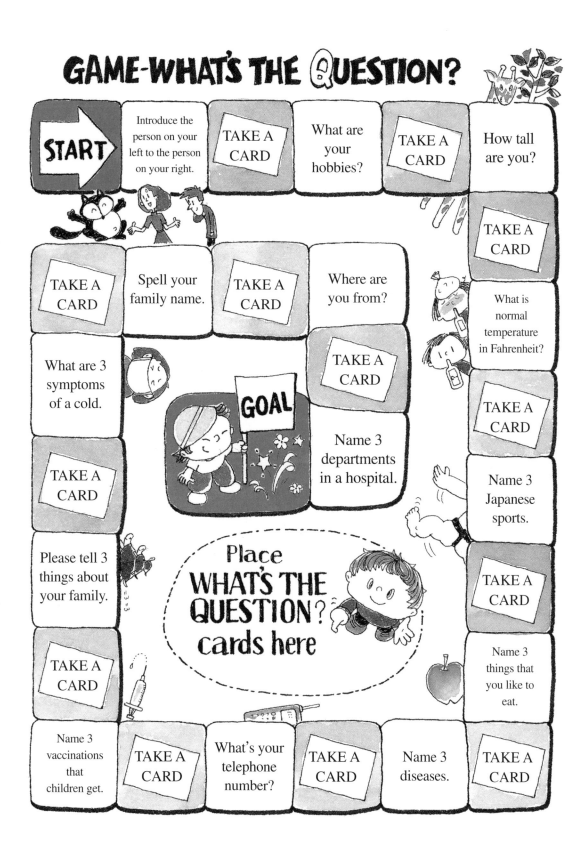

START

Introduce the person on your left to the person on your right.

TAKE A CARD

What are your hobbies?

TAKE A CARD

How tall are you?

TAKE A CARD

TAKE A CARD

Spell your family name.

TAKE A CARD

Where are you from?

What is normal temperature in Fahrenheit?

What are 3 symptoms of a cold.

TAKE A CARD

GOAL

TAKE A CARD

Name 3 departments in a hospital.

TAKE A CARD

Name 3 Japanese sports.

TAKE A CARD

Please tell 3 things about your family.

Place WHAT'S THE QUESTION? cards here

TAKE A CARD

TAKE A CARD

Name 3 things that you like to eat.

Name 3 vaccinations that children get.

TAKE A CARD

What's your telephone number?

TAKE A CARD

Name 3 diseases.

TAKE A CARD

119

Glossary

120

influenza (flu)　インフルエンザ, 流行性感冒　43

inhale　（息などを）吸い込む　52, 59

injection　注射　cf. shot　72, 98, 102

injure　けがをさせる, 傷つける　cf. hurt　49

injury　傷害, けが　67

inoculation　予防接種　63, 72-74, 76, 81, 82

inpatient　入院患者　cf. outpatient　85

insert　挿入する　50, 53, 57, 58, 87, 89, 92-94, 102, 104

insulin　インスリン　115, 117

insurance card　保険証　16, 17

intercourse (sexual intercourse)　性交　65, 69

internal examination (exam)　内診　63, 66

internal medicine (department of —)　内科　11, 12

internal use medicine　内服薬　104

internist　内科医　12

interval　間隔　73, 77

intestinal　腸の　85, 94, 96

intestine(s)　腸　96

large intestine　大腸　91

small intestine　小腸　91

introduce　紹介する　9, 36, 119

irregular　不規則な　61, 69

irritable bowel syndrome　過敏性腸症候群　43

Islamic　イスラム教徒（の）　109, 112

itch　かゆい, かゆみを生じさせる　108

itchy　かゆい　23

item　品物, 事項　86, 88, 92-94

IUD (intrauterine device)　避妊リング　61, 62, 66

IV (intravenous) drip　点滴　34, 87, 89, 93, 94

J

Japanese encephalitis　日本脳炎　72, 76, 77

jaundice　黄疸　64, 66

Jehovah's Witness　エホバの証人　108, 109, 114

Jewish　ユダヤ人の, ユダヤ教徒（の）　48, 108-110, 112

Judaism　ユダヤ教　114

K

kidney　腎臓　43, 90, 91

kidney stone　腎結石　43

kin　親族　38, 39

next of kin　最近親者　39

Korean　朝鮮（韓国）（人）の, 朝鮮（韓国）人　111, 114

kosher food　ユダヤ教の法にかなった（清浄な）食べ物　110

L

lab technician　検査技師　11

labor　分娩, 陣痛　66

labor room　分娩室, 陣痛室　63, 64, 66

latex glove(s)　ゴム手袋　34

laundry　洗濯もの, 洗濯場　32, 33

laxative　下剤　54, 86

lens　レンズ　50

lethargic　だるい, 無気力な　23, 75

leukemia　白血病　43, 45

lightly　そっと, 少しばかり　104

lining　裏, 内層　53, 71

liquid meal　流動食　54, 86, 88, 93

listen to (heart, lungs)　（心臓, 肺の）音を聞く　59, 96, 102

live birth　生児出生, 生産　62, 66

liver　肝臓　39, 43, 90, 91

local (regional) anesthesia　局部（局所）麻酔　84, 85, 90, 94

lower back　腰　16, 22, 106

lower GI series (barium enema)　下部消化管造影（バリウム注腸）　53-55

low-salt　低塩の　38

lumbar puncture　腰椎穿刺　55

lump　腫れ物, しこり　16, 22

lung　肺　43, 90, 91

lung function　肺機能（検査）　50, 55

M

magnetic　磁気の　55, 57

mastectomy　乳房切除　90, 92, 94

maternal　母の　63

Maternal and Child Health Handbook　母子健康手帳　63, 72

maternity　母性, 出産の, 妊婦の　63, 66

measles　麻疹, はしか　72, 73, 76, 77, 79, 81

medical　医学の, 医療の, 内科の　10, 21, 75

medical chart　カルテ　34

medical history　病歴　46

medication　薬剤, 与薬　40-42, 76, 96, 104, 105, 110, 117

medicine　①薬, 薬剤, ②医学　cf. drug　11, 41, 52, 53, 104

take medicine　薬を服用する　104

menopause　閉経期, 更年期　62, 66

menstruate　月経がある　60-62, 66, 69

microscope　顕微鏡　34, 57

midwife　助産師　11, 12, 66, 114

miscarriage　流産　62, 66, 69

mold　かび　40, 48, 82

morning sickness　早朝嘔吐, つわり　66

morphine　モルヒネ　108

mosquito　蚊　76

MRI (magnetic resonance imaging)　磁気共鳴画像法　50, 55

124

126

1. 訳語は原則として本書で使われている意味だけを示した．
2. 通常の辞書の形式に従って単数形での表記を基本としたが，underpants のように複数形でしか使われないものは複数形のままとし，bowel(s) のように基本的には複数形で用いられることが多いが単数形もあり得るものには (s) をつけた．本文の Medical Terms では文脈を考慮し，語によっては複数形のまま表記した．
3. Activity 1 で読み上げられる単語（本文には表記がない単語）も含まれている．

Transcripts and Answers

Unit 1 Do you work on the surgical ward?

Activity 1 Listening Practice ⟨Audio 2⟩

1. Kenji: Could you tell me your name please?

   Delores: My name is Delores Agosto.

   Kenji: Could you spell your first name please?

   Delores: D-E-L-O-R-E-S.

   Kenji: And could you spell your family name?

   Delores: A-G-O-S-T-O.

   Kenji: Could you speak more slowly?

   Delores: Sure, A-G-O-S-T-O.

   A: c) Agosto

2. Yoko: Where do you live?

   Mr. Green: I live in Akasaka. Do you want my address?

   Yoko: No, but I would like your phone number.

   Mr. Green: It's 03-4952-8614.

   Yoko: Could you say that again please?

   Mr. Green: 03-4952-8614.

   Yoko: Did you say 8641 or 8614?

   Mr. Green: I said 8614.

   A: a) 03-4952-8614

3. Mariko: What do you do?

   Enrique: I'm talking with you.

   Mariko: No, I mean, what's your occupation?

   Enrique: I'm sorry, what is the meaning of occupation?

   Mariko: It means job. What is your job?

   Enrique: Oh, I'm an X-ray technician.

   A: b) She wants to know his occupation.

4. Eli: Dr. Fujimoto, this is Harvey Jones. He's a nurse in the psychiatric department. Harvey, this is Dr. Kimie Fujimoto. She's an obstetrician.

   Harvey: How do you do?

   Dr. Fujimoto: It's really nice to meet you.

   Harvey: I'm sorry, I didn't get your name, doctor.

   Dr. Fujimoto: It's Kimie Fujimoto. My family name is spelled F-U-J-I-M-O-T-O.

   Harvey: I see. Thank you.

   A: b) He's a nurse.

Activity 3 Dialog ⟨Audio 4⟩

1. introduce	8. show you the ropes
2. How do you do	9. are you from
3. Please don't hesitate	10. nursing school
4. rounds	11. you are my senior
5. nurses' lounge	12. near this hospital
6. This is	13. hobbies
7. ward	14. great idea

Activity 4 Puzzle

1. OBSTETRICS	9. OPHTHALMOLOGY
2. INTERNAL MEDICINE	10. REHABILITATION
3. DENTISTRY	11. PSYCHIATRY
4. PEDIATRICS	12. DERMATOLOGY
5. RADIOLOGY	13. ANESTHESIOLOGY
6. GYNECOLOGY	14. ORTHOPEDICS
7. CARDIOLOGY	15. NEUROLOGY
8. PLASTIC SURGERY	16. ORAL SURGERY

Unit 2 What's your problem today?

Activity 1 Listening Practice ⟨Audio 5⟩

1. Masako: Is this your first visit?

   Mr. Wong: Yes, it is.

   Masako: Do you have an insurance card?

   Mr. Wong: No, I don't.

   Masako: What department do you want to visit?

   Mr. Wong: Well, I'm suffering from lower back pain, so I think I should go to the orthopedics department.

   A: b) He's got lower back pain.

2. Masako: What's your problem today, Mrs. Jefferson?

   Mrs. Jefferson: I've been feeling sick for two days.

   Masako: What are your symptoms?

   Mrs. Jefferson: I have a cough and diarrhea.

   Masako: Do you have a fever?

   Mrs. Jefferson: Yes, my temperature is 38℃.

   A: b) She has a fever, diarrhea and a cough.

3. Masako: What department would you like to visit?

   Ms. Goldberg: Well, I'm not sure.

   Masako: What seems to be the problem?

   Ms. Goldberg: I found a lump in my breast.

   Masako: Then, I think you had better go to the surgical department.

   A: b) Surgery

4. Masako: Mr. Jones, how have you been feeling?

Mr. Jones: I haven't been feeling well recently.

Masako: What's the matter?

Mr. Jones: I've had stomach pain and heartburn.

Masako: How long have you had these symptoms?

Mr. Jones: I've been having pain for about two months and I often get heartburn in the evening.

Masako: Have you had any nausea or vomiting?

Mr. Jones: Yes, this past week I've been nauseous every day.

A: c) For two months.

Activity 3 Dialog ⟨Audio 7⟩

1. Have you visited	8. suffering from
2. fill in this form	9. How long
3. Could you spell	10. about 3 or 4
4. height	11. Almost every day
5. weigh	12. with your heart
6. I'm 55 years old	13. when I was a patient
7. your problem	14. will see you

Activity 4 Puzzle

9, 8, 3, 11, 4, 7, 2, 6, 1, 10, 5

Unit 3 This is the nurses' station.

Activity 1 Listening Practice ⟨Audio 8⟩

1. Masako: Visiting hours are from 1 to 7 on weekdays and from 11 to 7 on Saturdays and Sundays.

Mr. Martin: I see. What time is lunch served?

Masako: At 12 o'clock noon.

A: c) from 11 to 7

2. Masako: This is the bath. Men can use it on Monday, Wednesday and Friday and women can use it on Tuesday, Thursday and Saturday.

Mr. Martin: Can I take a bath this morning?

Masako: No, the hours are from 2 to 5 in the afternoon. You will need to take a bath before your surgery or before some tests. A nurse will tell you when you can use it.

A: c) Tuesday, Thursday, Saturday

3. Mr. Martin: Can I eat my meals in my own room?

Masako: Patients who can walk should go to the dining room for their meals. After surgery or if you need rest, your meals will be brought to your room.

Mr. Martin: What time are the meals?

Masako: Breakfast is at 7:30 am, lunch at 12 noon and din-

ner at 6 pm.

A: c) dining room

4. Masako: This is the nurse call button by your bed. If you need a nurse's assistance, please push this button. There is also a nurse call button in the bath and in the toilet.

Mr. Martin: Where is the toilet?

Masako: It's down the hall on the left.

A: c) toilet, bath, patient's bed

Activity 3 Dialog ⟨Audio 10⟩

1. nurse	8. Across from
2. head nurse	9. in the lobby
3. clothes	10. The toilets are
4. bedside table	11. wash your face
5. change into your pajamas	12. What's in this room
6. around the ward	13. from 9 am to 6 pm
7. nurses' station	14. on your left

Activity 4 Puzzle 1

A: examination room

B: laundry

C: dining room

D: consultation room

E: bath

Activity 4 Puzzle 2

(23)	baby bottle	(5)	nurse call button
(11)	bedpan	(9)	oxygen
(4)	blood pressure gauge	(25)	scale
(7)	cast	(6)	sling
(8)	crutches	(3)	spouted water cup
(22)	diaper	(21)	stethoscope
(2)	emesis (kidney) basin	(24)	stretcher
(20)	examination table	(15)	syringe (needle)
(1)	gauze	(13)	thermometer
(10)	IV drip	(19)	vital signs monitor
(14)	latex gloves	(12)	walker
(18)	medical chart	(17)	X-ray
(16)	microscope		

Unit 4 Are you suffering from any illnesses?

Activity 1 Listening Practice ⟨Audio 11⟩

1. Masako: Ms. Cane, could you tell me your next of kin or

someone we can contact in case of emergency?

Ms. Cane: Masayoshi Kitano.

Masako: What's his relationship to you?

Ms. Cane: He's my husband.

Masako: Could you tell me his phone number at work and at home?

Ms. Cane: Our home number is 4381‐6517 and his work number is 5873‐4632.

A: c) He is Ms. Cane's husband.

2. Masako: What is your regular diet, Ms. Cane?

Ms. Cane: Well, I eat 3 meals a day, plus a snack in the afternoon. I try to eat a balanced diet.

Masako: Do you have any restrictions in your diet?

Ms. Cane: Yes, I eat a low-salt diet because of my hypertension.

Masako: I see. Do you eat rice at every meal?

Ms. Cane: I eat rice once or twice a day.

A: b) She doesn't eat very salty food.

3. Masako: Do you smoke?

Ms. Cane: Now, I don't. But I used to smoke. I smoked for 7 years, but I quit 2 years ago.

Masako: Do you drink alcohol?

Ms. Cane: A little. I drink a glass of wine or beer every day.

A: b) She drinks a glass every day.

4. Masako: Could you tell me your family history? Are your parents alive?

Ms. Cane: My mother is alive. She suffers from diabetes. My father passed away 5 years ago. He had a heart attack. I have a younger brother and older sister. My sister also has hypertension. My brother is healthy.

Masako: Do you have any children?

Ms. Cane: Yes, I have 2 daughters, age 19 and 23 and a son, age 17.

A: a) He had a heart attack.

Activity 3 Dialog ⟨Audio 13⟩

1. hospital
2. admission
3. my right side
4. hypertension
5. suffering from
6. Have you ever
7. I'm taking
8. your doctor
9. allergies
10. daily activities
11. bathtub
12. vision and hearing
13. personality
14. worried about
15. can speak English

Activity 4 Puzzle

U	A	A	C	A	T	A	R	A	C	T	Q	R	E	A
W	X	S	P	L	E	U	K	E	M	I	A	S	M	F
H	L	E	T	P	K	S	S	N	A	A	A	E	F	X
S	A	P	T	H	E	A	E	D	B	E	Z	D	R	E
I	S	I	B	U	M	N	H	Y	S	C	B	U	A	E
S	I	L	R	B	O	A	D	I	E	Y	X	P	C	N
O	T	E	E	V	B	G	D	I	Q	X	V	A	T	O
L	I	P	D	A	L	T	A	V	C	R	M	J	U	T
U	L	S	E	H	R	I	J	M	D	I	B	M	R	S
C	L	Y	V	A	D	P	O	L	P	S	T	L	E	L
R	I	G	E	S	C	B	M	T	L	Z	E	I	Y	L
E	S	H	D	I	A	B	E	T	E	S	P	V	S	A
B	N	H	E	P	A	T	I	T	I	S	L	U	I	G
U	O	K	M	M	S	I	L	O	H	O	C	L	A	H
T	T	L	N	O	I	S	N	E	T	R	E	P	Y	H

1. 喘息
2. 後天性免疫不全症候群（エイズ）
3. アルコール依存症
4. 虫垂炎
5. 白内障
6. 糖尿病
7. 湿疹
8. てんかん
9. 骨折
10. 胆石
11. 痛風
12. 心臓病
13. 肝炎
14. じん麻疹
15. 高血圧（症）
16. 白血病
17. 扁桃炎
18. 結核

Unit 5 **You need to have an MRI.**

Activity 1 Listening Practice ⟨Audio 14⟩

1. Masako: I need to take a blood sample, Ms. Smith.

   Ms. Smith: All right.

   Masako: Could you please put your arm here and make a fist. OK, you can relax now. Have you ever had any problems with your blood clotting?

   Ms. Smith: No, I haven't.

   Masako: OK, please apply pressure for 3 minutes.

   A: b) taking a blood sample.

2. Masako: Mr. Silver, before your surgery, you need to have a blood test, urine test, lung function test and an ECG.

   Mr. Silver: Should I have the tests today or after I'm admitted?

   Masako: You should have the tests after your admission.

   A: d) after his admission

3. Masako: Ms. Jackson, your doctor said you need to have a gastroscopy.

   Ms. Jackson: I never had one before. What is it?

   Masako: The doctor inserts a long tube with a lens into your stomach through your mouth. He can examine your stomach with it.

   Ms. Jackson: I see.

   A: b) her stomach

4. Masako: Mr. Kim, you need to have an RI. Please take this elevator to the first floor. Turn right and go to the X-ray department; that's window 30.

   Mr. Kim: I should go to the first floor, then turn right and go to window 30.

   Masako: Yes, that's right. Just give them this form.

   A: a) an RI

Activity 3 Dialog ⟨Audio 16⟩

1. some tests	7. about the test
2. X-ray	8. lining
3. chest	9. need to have
4. your stomach	10. take your temperature
5. a little	11. tomorrow morning
6. be painful	12. Please take

Activity 4 Crossword Puzzle

ACROSS

1. URINALYSIS

5. BLOOD TEST

7. ECHOGRAM

10. BARIUM ENEMA

12. EYE TEST

DOWN

2. BLOOD PRESSURE TEST

3. ELECTROCARDIOGRAM

4. CT SCAN

6. ENDOSCOPY

8. X-RAY

9. BIOPSY

11. MRI

Unit 6 **You're going to have a baby!**

Activity 1 Listening Practice ⟨Audio 17⟩

1. Mariko: What's the purpose of your visit?

   Mary: I think I'm pregnant.

   Mariko: When was your last period?

   Mary: About 6 weeks ago.

   Mariko: OK, we'll give you a pregnancy test.

   A: b) She wants a pregnancy test.

2. Mariko: What's your problem today, Sarah?

   Sarah: I'm pregnant and I want to have an abortion.

   Mariko: Did you have a pregnancy test?

   Sarah: Yes, I did a home pregnancy test and it was positive.

   A: c) Her home pregnancy test was positive.

3. Mariko: When did you start menstruating?

   Susan: When I was 12 years old.

   Mariko: When was your last period?

   Susan: It began 2 weeks ago, on May 17th.

   A: c) She was 12 years old.

4. Ms. Grimes: I'd like to be tested for HIV.

   Mariko: All right, just take a number and wait for a few minutes.

   Ms. Grimes: When can I get the results of the test?

   Mariko: Come back in one week. Don't forget to bring your number.

   A: b) She wants an HIV test.

Activity 3 Dialog 〈Audio 19〉

1. to have a baby	8. before and after
2. Please bring it with you	9. its color is
3. kinds of tests	10. good for the baby
4. Every 5 minutes	11. sleep most
5. labor	12. if your baby has any
6. Let's go to	problems
7. push harder	

Activity 6 Crossword Puzzle

ACROSS

3. D & C
6. LABOR
7. MORNING SICKNESS
8. FETUS
10. ABORTION
12. PILL
13. CERVIX
14. DELIVERY
15. PAP SMEAR
17. BIRTH CONTROL

DOWN

1. VAGINA
2. PLACENTA
4. CONTRACTIONS
5. CESAREAN SECTION
7. MISCARRIAGE
9. MIDWIFE
11. UTERUS
16. APGAR SCORE

Unit 7 My baby has a fever.

Activity 1 Listening Practice 〈Audio 20〉

1. Akari: What's Mary's problem today?

    Mrs. Arthur: I think she has a stomach virus.

    Akari: What are her symptoms?

    Mrs. Arthur: She's been vomiting and has diarrhea.

    Akari: How long has she had these symptoms?

    Mrs. Arthur: Since around noon yesterday.

    Akari: Does she have a fever?

    Mrs. Arthur: Yes, her temperature was 38.7°C this morning.

    Akari: Let's check her temperature now, please put this thermometer under her armpit.

    A: c) for 1 day

2. Akari: Hello, Mrs. Fisher. How is Howard feeling today?

    Mrs. Fisher: He's very fine. We're here for his DPT booster.

    Akari: When did he have his first shot?

    Mrs. Fisher: It's right here in the Maternal and Child Health Handbook. A little over a year ago.

    Akari: Does he have a fever or has he been feeling sick this past week?

    Mrs. Fisher: No, he's been very healthy recently.

    A: b) over a year ago

3. Akari: Ms. Ryan, what's the matter with your daughter?

    Ms. Ryan: She fell and hit her head.

    Akari: How far did she fall?

    Ms. Ryan: About a meter.

    Akari: Has she had any unusual symptoms, like vomiting?

    Ms. Ryan: No, she didn't vomit.

    Akari: OK. Just wait here and we'll X-ray her head right away.

    A: b) She hit her head.

4. Akari: What is the purpose of your visit today?

    Mr. Jones: I'd like my son, Alan, to have a vaccination.

    Akari: What kind of vaccination does he need?

    Mr. Jones: I'd like him to have an MMR vaccination.

    Akari: We don't give measles, mumps and rubella in one injection in Japan. He'll have to have each one separately.

    Mr. Jones: I see. So what should I do?

    Akari: Why don't we give him the measles vaccine today and you can come back for the other two vaccinations.

    Mr. Jones: OK. That's what I'll do.

    A: c) Measles, mumps and rubella

Activity 3 Dialog 〈Audio 22〉

1. My son is	7. is suffering from
2. to be the problem	8. you can mix it
3. his ear	9. If you have any questions
4. under his armpit	10. What else
5. have any allergies	11. other inoculations
6. does have a fever	12. What's that

Activity 4 Puzzle

E	M	M	I	P	S	E	L	S	A	E	M
D	N	U	M	O	R	N	U	D	X	O	O
I	P	C	M	R	W	N	E	L	G	I	C
P	S	T	E	P	S	O	D	B	L	H	X
H	I	E	U	P	S	T	I	O	H	L	L
T	S	T	M	Z	H	F	P	C	X	X	F
H	S	A	J	D	O	A	K	O	A	X	X
E	U	N	G	Y	D	E	L	A	X	A	H
R	T	U	P	P	N	C	G	I	G	T	Q
I	R	S	T	P	N	L	J	I	T	C	U
A	E	G	O	F	A	D	W	J	D	I	B
J	P	X	V	A	L	L	E	B	U	R	S

3. 百日咳
4. 風疹
5. 水疱瘡
6. おたふくかぜ
7. ポリオ
8. 破傷風
9. ジフテリア
10. 麻疹

Unit 8 Your surgery will be tomorrow at 10 am.

Activity 1 Listening Practice ⟨Audio 23⟩

1. Mr. Edwards: What kind of surgery do I need?

   Masako: You need to have a hernia removed from your abdomen, Mr. Edwards.

   Mr. Edwards: How long will I have to stay in the hospital?

   Masako: About two weeks. First, you need to have tests, then you need about a week for your recovery from the surgery.

   A: a) one week

2. Masako: Ms. Smith, how are you doing today?

   Ms. Smith: I'm nervous about my gallbladder operation.

   Masako: Gallbladder surgery is one of the easiest operations. These days the surgeon does it using a camera making just 3 small slits. The recovery time is very quick and there is little post-op pain.

   Ms. Smith: I'm relieved to hear that.

   A: c) gallbladder surgery

3. Mr. Horowitz: I'm having anal surgery tomorrow, and I'm wondering what kind of anesthesia they'll use.

Masako: The anesthesiologist will come and talk to you later about your anesthesia, Mr. Horowitz.

   Mr. Horowitz: Do you think they'll use general anesthesia? I don't want to be awake during my operation.

   Masako: These days they use many kinds of anesthesia, general, epidural, spinal, local. But don't worry! They'll use general anesthesia so you'll be asleep when they perform your operation.

   A: a) general anesthesia

4. Masako: Ms. Cotto, you need to prepare some things before your surgery.

   Ms. Cotto: What kinds of things?

   Masako: You need some towels, a toothbrush and toothpaste and 2 paper shopping bags.

   Ms. Cotto: That's a lot of things; let me write it down. OK, anything else?

   Masako: Yes, for breast surgery, you also need a gown which opens in the front, 1 cotton T-binder, a pair of underpants, 2 chest binders, a pair of pajamas and a spouted water cup.

   Ms. Cotto: Where can I get these things?

   Masako: At the hospital shop. Just show them this list.

   Ms. Cotto: Oh, that's very convenient.

   A: b) at the hospital shop

Activity 3 Dialog ⟨Audio 26⟩

1. Wednesday morning
2. shopping bags
3. write your name
4. your doctor will talk with you
5. take a bath
6. You can drink water
7. Please go to the toilet
8. remove your watch
9. operating room
10. lie on your left side
11. your surgery is over

Activity 4 Puzzle

appendix（虫垂）27

bladder（膀胱）20

bone（骨）9

brain（脳）8

duodenum（十二指腸）19

esophagus（食道）11

gallbladder（胆嚢）16

heart（心臓）29

kidney（腎臓）24

large intestine（大腸）28

liver（肝臓）6

lung（肺）1

ovary（卵巣）10

pancreas（膵臓）21

penis（陰茎）3

prostate（前立腺）13

rectum（直腸）22

rib（肋骨）25

small intestine（小腸）2

spleen（脾臓）17

stomach（胃）7

testicle（精巣，睾丸）23

throat（喉）26

thyroid（甲状腺）15

tonsil（扁桃腺）4

ureter（尿管）18

uterus（子宮）5

uvula（口蓋垂）14

vagina（腟）12

Unit 9 How are you feeling?

Activity 1 Listening Practice 〈Audio 27〉

1. Masako: Mr. Jones, how are you feeling today?

   Mr. Jones: I'm not feeling so good.

   Masako: What's the matter?

   Mr. Jones: I couldn't sleep very well last night.

   Masako: Are you feeling any pain?

   Mr. Jones: Yes, my abdominal area is very painful.

   Masako: It's probably gas. Let me listen to your intestines.
   Yes, you have a lot of intestinal movement. Getting out of bed and walking will help you get rid of the gas.
   A: b) He has gas.

2. Masako: Good morning, Ms. Appleby. How are you feeling?

   Ms. Appleby: I'm feeling pretty good.

   Masako: What's your temperature?

   Ms. Appleby: It's 37°C.

   Masako: How was your appetite yesterday?

Ms. Appleby: It was good. I ate about $\frac{3}{4}$ of my meals.
   A: c) She ate 75%.

3. Masako: Good morning, Maribel. How are you feeling today?

   Maribel: Good morning, Ms. Sato. I'm feeling fine.

   Masako: Maribel, yesterday, how many times did you move your bowels?

   Maribel: I don't understand "bowels."

   Masako: It means number two. How many times did you do number two?

   Maribel: Let me see, 3 times.

   Masako: OK, and how many times did you urinate?

   Maribel: Does that mean number one?

   Masako: Yes.

   Maribel: I did number one, I think 6 times.
   A: a) 6 times.

4. Masako: How are you feeling today, Ms. Silverstein?

   Ms. Silverstein: I'm feeling much better.

   Masako: I'm glad to hear that. I need to take your blood pressure.

   Ms. Silverstein: How is my blood pressure?

   Masako: It's good. It's 130 over 84. Here's your medication. This is for one day.

   Ms. Silverstein: When should I take it?

   Masako: Please take 2 yellow tablets and 1 pink capsule, 3 times a day after meals.

   Ms. Silverstein: I take 2 yellow tablets and 1 pink capsule, 3 times a day after meals.

   Masako: Yes, that's right.
   A: d) 3 times a day after meals

Activity 3 Dialog 〈Audio 29〉

1. Where am I	7. The doctor will
2. your temperature	8. may feel dizzy
3. I have something	9. sit up slowly
4. brush your teeth	10. to your beds
5. I have some pain	11. in five days
6. feeling much better	12. your medicine

Activity 4 Puzzle

Scrambled Sentences

1. Your drip is finished.

2. I'm going to take a blood sample.

3. I'm going to insert a suppository into your anus.

4. Please change into this surgical gown.

5. Please take your temperature.

6. Your blood pressure is 150 over 85.

7. I'm going to give you an enema.

8. Do you need to use the bedpan?

9. I need to give you an injection.

10. I have to change the dressing on your wound.

11. The doctor will remove your stitches tomorrow.

12. Take the elevator to the first floor.

13. Please put a urine sample in this cup.

14. I want to listen to your lungs.

15. Do you feel nauseous?

16. Please call a nurse if you need to go to the toilet.

(If you need to go to the toilet, please call a nurse)

Matching

A) 8	E) 5	I) 12	M) 14
B) 3	F) 15	J) 1	N) 9
C) 11	G) 10	K) 13	O) 7
D) 16	H) 4	L) 6	P) 2

Unit 10 Are you worried about anything?

Activity 1 Listening Practice 〈Audio 30〉

1. Yuko: Hello, Mrs. Lieberman, I'm Yuko Tanaka. I'm going to be your nurse.

Mrs. Lieberman: Oh, hello.

Yuko: I want to ask you if you have any dietary restrictions.

Mrs. Lieberman: Well, I'm Jewish, so I'm not allowed to eat any pork or shellfish.

Yuko: I'll let our dietitian know about your request.

Mrs. Lieberman: Thank you very much. I was worried about the meals here.

A: c) She can't eat shellfish and pork.

2. Akari: Good morning, Billy.

Billy: Good morning, Ms. Fujii.

Akari: How are you feeling?

Billy: I feel OK, but my stitches itch.

Akari: That means you're healing well. The doctor will take out your stitches soon.

Billy: Does it hurt when the doctor takes out the stitches?

Akari: Just a tiny bit.

A: d) He's worried it will hurt when the doctor takes out his stitches.

3. Masako: Mrs. Jennings, do you have any concerns about your hospital admission?

Mrs. Jennings: I need to have heart surgery, and I'm worried about needing a blood transfusion.

Masako: Well, there is some possibility you may need a transfusion during surgery.

Mrs. Jennings: I can't have a blood transfusion. I'm a Jehovah's Witness. Jehovah's Witnesses aren't allowed to have blood transfusions.

Masako: I see. Why don't we talk about your wishes together with your husband and your doctor?

A: c) Because of her religion.

4. Masako: Good morning, Mr. Philips. How are you feeling today?

Mr. Philips: I'm feeling a lot of pain.

Masako: I'm sorry to hear that. I'll talk to your doctor about increasing your painkillers.

Mr. Philips: Thank you. I'd appreciate that.

Masako: Do you have any other concerns or worries?

Mr. Philips: Well, my cancer is getting worse. I'm worried about the pain. I'm afraid that my doctor won't give me enough painkillers.

Masako: Please, don't worry about that. We'll do everything we can to keep you comfortable.

A: a) He wants more painkillers.

Activity 3 Dialog 〈Audio 32〉

1. Welcome to this hospital

2. first visit

3. foreign patients

4. there are differences

5. special needs of

6. the main difference

7. The other thing

8. a person's religion

9. he'd be happy

10. nurse visiting from

11. Are you having any problems

12. I'm worried about

13. I can help explain

14. a chance to talk

15. didn't realize

Activity 4 Puzzle

1. c	2. b	3. a, b, c	4. c	5. a
6. b	7. b	8. b, c	9. c	10. c